Recognizing
Alcoholism
and Its Effects

Harvey R. St. Clair

Recognizing Alcoholism and Its Effects

A Mini-Guide

KARGER

Basel · München · Paris · London · New York ·
New Delhi · Bangkok · Singapore · Tokyo · Sydney

About the Author

Dr. St. Clair was formerly the Clinical Director of the Substance Abuse Treatment Program, Our Lady of Peace Hospital, Louisville, Ky. He is currently the Director of the Alcohol Treatment Program, Veterans Administration Medical Center, Louisville, Ky. He is certified by the American Society of Addiction Medicine. Formerly Clinical Professor, he is currently Associate Professor, Department of Psychiatry and Behavioral Science, School of Medicine, University of Louisville, Ky.

Library of Congress Cataloging-in-Publication Data
    St. Clair, Harvey R., 1921–
    Recognizing alcoholism and its effects. A mini-guide / Harvey R. St. Clair.
    Includes bibliographical references and index.
    1. Alcoholism. 2. Alcohol – Toxicology. I. Title.
    [DNLM: 1. Alcohol, Ethyl – adverse affects. 2. Alcoholism.]
    ISBN 3–8055–5395–1

Drug Dosage

    The author and the publisher have exerted every effort to ensure that drug selection and dosage set forth in this text are in accord with current recommendations and practice at the time of publication. However, in view of ongoing research, changes in government regulations, and the constant flow of information relating to drug therapy and drug reactions, the reader is urged to check the package insert for each drug for any change in indications and dosage and for added warnings and precautions. This is particularly important when the recommended agent is a new and/or infrequently employed drug.

©   Copyright 1991 by S. Karger AG, P.O. Box, CH–4009 Basel (Switzerland)
    Printed in Switzerland on acid-free paper by Thür AG Offsetdruck, Pratteln
    ISBN 3–8055–5395–1

Dedicated to *Bill Emonz*

Contents

Preface

Alcoholism is the most frequently missed diagnosis in medical care, the object of the greatest prejudice, and the most frequently mismanaged illness in treatment. Alcoholism is the third most important public health problem in the US, ranking behind only cardiovascular diseases and cancer, yet it is the most neglected topic in medical school and postgraduate training. Steps to correct these training deficits have recently begun to be taken. This synopsis is intended primarily for use by medical students and house staff, yet it may also prove useful to those who missed more detailed training in alcoholism, as well as other interested professionals and lay persons.

This is not a textbook. There is ample literature available in the field for those who wish to learn more. The references will provide further reading.

1   History

Alcoholic beverages have been made since prerecorded history and are still being made by even remote tribes and Stone Age level peoples. Meads from honey, wines from fruits, and beer from cereals were the first. Distillation of spirits was discovered about 800 AD by an Arabian, Zeber. The word alcohol is Arabic and means 'finely divided spirit'. Alcoholism was first identified as a disease by Benjamin Rush, the father of American psychiatry, in 1786. The Alcoholics Anonymous movement began in the late 1930s. The field existed as a step-child in medicine until the psychiatrists, Harry Tiebout and Ruth Fox, subspecialized in it in the 1950s. It has only been in the last decade and a half that the American Medical Association and the American Psychiatric Association have urged much more emphasis on alcoholism in committees, in curricula and in subspecialization. The American Medical Society on Alcoholism and Other Drug Dependencies and the American Academy of Psychiatrists in Alcoholism and Addictions are recently established organizations devoted to the field.

Alcohol abuse and dependency are highly stigmatized in human behaviors. Intoxication is socially unacceptable (except perhaps for some groups of adolescents) and has social and legal consequences. In the US we still jail people for public intoxication. We still call people 'drunks' in a derogatory sense. The concept of it being a disease was recently rejected by the US Supreme Court for Veterans Administration benefits purposes. A majority, including many otherwise enlightened, still consider it a moral or characterologic weakness.

Many religions consider it sinful, and contribute further to guilt identifications. The prejudices and misconceptions about it are ubiquitous. The only hope of correcting these inaccuracies and prejudices lies in education with scientific data. Unfortunately, this educational process is in its embryonic state.

2 Epidemiology, Morbidity and Mortality

The exact prevalence is hard to study, but the figures quoted are reasonable. Regier at NIMH collected data in 1984 that indicated the national average of alcohol diagnoses to be 7–8 % of the general population. Figures often quoted are 10 % of adult males and 5 % of adult females with the disease, but these figures are converging. A lifetime prevalence of 19 % for males has been recently identified. Other figures are that 30 % of US adult males are heavy drinkers; 25–50 % of young males have alcohol-related problems; 25–50 % of the young have transient alcohol-related problems; 20–35 % of male medical/surgical hospitalized patients are alcoholic (with the diagnosis very frequently missed); and alcohol is related to 10 % of all deaths in the US per year. Alcoholism consumes 12 % of all health expenditures and 20 % of all hospital costs. Over two thirds of US males drink more than just occasionally. Prevalence is related to longevity with there being a U-shaped curve associated with longevity. The mean age of onset is 21 years for males.

Higher prevalence rates exist in the lower socioeconomic class, lower educational groups, single, urban WASPs, Irish and French Catholics, prisoners, and male homosexuals who frequent gay bars. Lower prevalence exists in Jews, Muslims, Mormons, Methodists, Southern Baptists and lesbians. There is a direct relationship between the number of alcohol arrests, the unemployed and those on welfare with the prevalence of alcoholism. There is also a positive correlation between the number of liquor stores per county and both deaths from drunken driving and prison population.

Continued abuse lowers longevity by approximately 15 years. Deaths are from cardiac disease, infections, accidents, suicide, liver disease, pancreatitis, cancer and other causes. Many conceptualize alcoholism itself as slow suicide. 15–20% of alcoholics suicide. Death from infections was found in 25% of alcoholics in one series. Traffic deaths are the fourth leading cause of death up to age 40 and alcohol is involved in approximately 50% of these. Incidentally, a blood alcohol level of 0.08% is sufficient to clearly impair driving ability, not the 0.10% states in most laws. At least 80% of those arrested for driving under the influence (DUI) are alcoholics. Alcohol abuse is a factor in almost 50% of all accidental deaths, suicides and homicides.

Various studies have resulted in varying statistics but at least 60% of alcoholics have at least another DSM-III-R, Axis I or II diagnosis. However, there is not a higher prevalence of alcoholism in schizophrenics, each diagnosis is coincidental, although there is a higher prevalence of both in the lower socio-economic class. There is a higher prevalence of antisocial and borderline personalities. Both sociopathy and alcoholism tend to burn out with age. Post-traumatic stress disorder predisposes to alcohol abuse.

More will be said later about subgroups such as women, adolescents, skid row, and dual diagnosis, since these involve psychodynamic issues.

Over 80% of the alcohol-abusing population are not getting treatment for it despite the marked increase in treatment facilities in recent years.

3 Diagnosis

Alcoholics seldom present as alcoholics except in emergency rooms. Most deny they are alcoholic and the vast majority minimize and lie about the amount. Denial is a hallmark of the disease.

There have been many definitions and classifications of alcoholism. The terms problem drinker and alcoholic are interchangeable. The alcoholisms are not a unitary disease but a heterogeneous group with varying degrees of severity, duration, consequences, progression and outcome. The groupings identified by Jellinek in 1960 (alpha, beta, gamma, delta, epsilon) are no longer valid, although still used today by some of the craft level professionals. There are many subgroups and subpopulations of alcoholics, each having their own features, but since nearly 400 of these have been identified it is not in the scope of this manual to elaborate on them. One useful concept that does have some validity is the division into primary and secondary, although this risks oversimplification. Primary is when the alcoholism came first and is independent of other, either coincidental or 'by-product' diseases, such as depression or cirrhosis. Secondary is when there is a pre-existing other disease, e.g., borderline personality disorder, bipolar disorder, PTSD, severe rheumatoid arthritis, etc., which has a causal link to alcohol abuse as a form of self-medication. The so-called types 1 and 2 need further study before being proven entities.

There have been more attempts in recent years to give a more exact definition of operational criteria. Research Diagnostic Criteria and the Diagnostic and Statistical Manual (DSM-III-R)

Michigan Alcoholism Screening Test

Questions	Answers with weighted scoring

1	Do you feel you are a normal drinker? (If patient denies any use of alcohol check here ___).	Yes ___ No _2_
2	Have you ever awakened the morning after some drinking the night before and found that you could not remember a part of the evening before?	Yes _2_ No ___
3	Does your spouse (or parents) ever worry or complain about your drinking?	Yes _1_ No ___
4	Can you stop drinking without a struggle after one or two drinks?	Yes ___ No _2_
5	Do you ever feel bad about your drinking?	Yes _1_ No ___
6	Do friends or relatives think you are a normal drinker?	Yes ___ No _2_
7	Do you ever try to limit your drinking to certain times of the day or to certain places?	Yes _0_ No ___
8	Are you always able to stop drinking when you want to?	Yes ___ No _2_
9	Have you ever attended a meeting of Alcoholics Anonymous (AA)?	Yes _5_ No ___
10	Have you gotten into fights when drinking?	Yes _1_ No ___
11	Has drinking ever created problems with you and your spouse?	Yes _2_ No ___
12	Has your spouse (or other family members) ever gone to anyone for help about your drinking?	Yes _2_ No ___
13	Have you ever lost friends or girlfriends because of drinking?	Yes _2_ No ___

Questions		Answers with weighted scoring
14	Have you ever gotten into trouble at work because of drinking?	Yes _2_ No___
15	Have you ever lost a job because of drinking?	Yes _2_ No___
16	Have you ever neglected your obligations, your family, or your work for 2 or more days in a row because you were drinking?	Yes _2_ No___
17	Do you ever drink before noon?	Yes _1_ No___
18	Have you ever been told you have liver trouble? Cirrhosis?	Yes _2_ No___
19	Have you ever had delirium tremens (DTs), severe shaking, heard voices, or seen things that were not there after heavy drinking?	Yes _2_ No___
20	Have you ever gone to anyone for help?	Yes _2_ No___
21	Have you ever been in a hospital because of your drinking?	Yes _5_ No___
22	Have you ever been a patient in a psychiatric hospital or on a psychiatric ward of a general hospital where drinking was part of the problem?	Yes _2_ No___
23	Have you ever been seen at a psychiatric or mental health clinic, or gone to a doctor, social worker, or clergyman for help with an emotional problem in which drinking had played a part?	Yes _2_ No___
24	Have you ever been arrested, even for a few hours, because of drunk behavior?	Yes _2_ No___
25	Have you ever been arrested for drunk driving or driving after drinking?	Yes _2_ No___

give quite acceptable diagnostic and classification criteria, but they will not be repeated here since these are readily available. The National Council on Alcoholism has separate physiological, dependency, organ pathology and behavioral criteria. Spitzer and Endicott have criteria for screening purposes that are quite similar to the Michigan Alcoholism Screening Test (MAST). The MAST is the most widely used and the most highly validated screening instrument and is copied here for convenience of use.

There is also the Short MAST Brief MAST for those who do not wish to take the 10 min to administer and score the MAST.

The MAST is most reliable when given to the spouse about the patient. Originally, MAST scores over 5 were considered pathological but many in the field consider scores of 5–9 highly suspicious and over 10 to be clearly significant. The MacAndrew scale, known as the 'MAC', is another useful screening device. This is a 49-item scale selected from the Minnesota Multiphasic Personality Inventory (MMPI) but with the caveat that if the F scale is 16 or more the scale is invalid. The CAGE questionnaire developed by Dr. John Ewing is also quite useful. It consists of only 4 salient questions: Have you ever felt you ought to cut down on your drinking? Have you been annoyed when others say you have had too much to drink? Have you ever felt bad or guilty about your drinking? Have you ever had a drink first thing in the morning to steady your nerves or get rid of a hangover (eye opener)? A score of 2 or more is positive. All of these are screening devices.

Alerting laboratory tests are especially a mean corpuscular volume of greater than 95–100 and a γ-glutamyltransferase (GGT) of greater than 85. Also commonly found are increased uric acid, elevated cholesterol and triglycerides, elevated liver enzymes and increased bilirubin. An unexplained elevation of fasting blood glucose is also suspicious in the absence of diabetes or a positive family history. Unexplained macrocytosis or macrocytic anemia are also suspicious.

Falls, tremors, fatigue, recent memory loss, cardiomyopathy, gastrointestinal tract bleeding, physical stigmata of ruddy face or nose, and a nontender enlarged liver raise the index of suspicion.

Psychosocial issues that should prompt further investigation are behavioral changes, anxiety, depression, serious losses, chronic severe emotional or physical stress, a DUI, a positive family history of alcoholism, or a steadily drinking peer group. Anxiety and depression are often produced by alcoholism. The diagnosis should not be just biological, but should use the biopsychosocial paradigm.

The author's own personal criteria for the diagnosis is that the person has crossed the boundary from social drinking to alcoholism when excessive drinking repeatedly leads to biological or psychological or sociological damage, whether the damage is transient or not.

Dr. Leo Kanner, when asked many years ago what determines when a person should seek professional help said, 'People have problems but when the problems have the people then is the time to go'.

4 Etiology, Risk Factors

Alcoholism has no single cause. Risk factors can be categorized into genetic, reward reinforcement, biological, sociocultural, behavioral, dynamic, ego strength, and stress paradigms. It is best to think of these as a heterogeneous polyglot of risk factors with different combinations and varying significance in each individual. The disease is a biopsychosocial one.

Heredity

Heritability is quite well accepted and heavily weighted as a risk factor. This is not to say, however, that the disease is inherited per se. The terminology is family history positive (FHP). If the siblings of the parents are included then the FHP prevalence is higher. Over 80% of both male and female alcoholics are FHP on one or both sides of the family. A certain number of alcoholics, however, are unaware of their FHP because of the diagnosis having been concealed. Monozygotic twins show an almost 100% concordance rate regardless of whether raised by their biologic or adoptive non-alcoholic families. Other adoptive studies irrefutably support genetic loading as a risk factor for males but are not as yet clear about females. FHP sons are four times as likely to develop alcoholism as family history negative sons. FHP offspring show higher levels of acetaldehyde and higher degrees of muscle relaxation with test doses of alcohol. FHP young males also show less intoxication and lowered amplitude and increased latency of the P300 on the EEG with test doses. FHP males become alcoholic at an earlier age and show more severity and progression than family history negative males. Monozygotic twins can consume greater quantities of alcohol than dizygotic twins. Finally, behavioral and pharmacologic reactions in both acute and chronic administration of alcohol in animals is heritable.

Reward Reinforcement

Alcohol produces an initial stimulating effect on the brain that is rewarding.WIn addition, the euphoric mood and disinhibition of impulses are ego syntonic. It is a common saying after extended effort or frustration for a person to say they 'need' a drink. There may even be some neurotransmitter stimulation of the reward centers in the brain. The isoquinolines and carbolines produced in the brain as by-products of alcohol metabolism are opiate-like. More will be discussed about these under the biology section. There is some evidence that the olfactory midbrain is involved in self-stimulation, suggesting primitive levels are involved.

Alcohol reduces dysphoria and/or enables the discharge of pent up emotions, both being ego syntonic and thus reward reinforcing.

Escape from stress, anxiety, tension, sorrow, loneliness, frustration, boredom, depression, etc., and overt mental illness is momentarily successful through alcohol. Feelings of helplessness, hopelessness, fear, panic, terror, anguish and loss of control, which can occur in many emotional crises, can be temporarily self-medicated with alcohol. Chronic pain can be numbed for awhile. Once these palliative measures are learned they are repetitively sought if the burdens continue.

If a person with a simple social phobia finds it melts with alcohol, or a shy person becomes socially comfortable, this becomes a reinforcement for repetition. Or if a person with suppressed and repressed anger can express it under the influence of alcohol, even inappropriately, the discharge of tension is rewarding.

Once there has been a sufficient number of instances of this conscious or unconscious self-medication for problems, then a pattern for chronic use may be established. Chronic use then becomes conditionally utilized for both abatement of dysphoria and seeking euphoria. At this point it ceases to be use but is abuse. While this level of abuse may not progress to alcoholism, it still becomes a problem unto itself. One remedy, of course, for this is to deny that it is a problem and to continue to drink. Many can control their drinking at this level and contain it without damage to self or others, but for others there is a progression to dependency. Those drinkers who use alcohol socially or before or during dinner with the family are still involved in reward reinforcement since it becomes a habit they look forward to with pleasure and are apt to continue it.

With chronic use there is the additional phenomenon of tolerance and this leads to using larger amounts of alcohol to achieve the desired effects. Social drinkers can usually resist tolerance and not escalate the amount they use. Social drinkers who do escalate over time should be identified as self-medicators or as addicted unless proven otherwise. Once escalation becomes an established routine the person is in the early stages of alcoholism.

Biologic

Although the final data are not yet in and the importance of these is speculative, nonetheless these research findings are most interesting and are currently enjoying wide publicity.

Acetaldehyde and catecholamines, especially dopamine, combine to make tetrahydroisoquinoline (THIQ); acetaldehyde and indolamines, 5-hydroxytryptophan (5HT) or tryptamine, combine to make tetrahydro-β-carbolines (Salsolinol); 3,4-dihydroxyphenyl-l-acetaldehyde combine with dopamine to form tetrahydropapaveroline (THP). These are all opiate-like alkaloids, THP is the precursor of the morphine alkaloids in the opium poppy. These bind to neuroamine receptors and act as false neurotransmitters. When given to rats there is a modest increase in voluntary intake of ETOH. Monkeys do not naturally prefer alcohol to water, yet when given THP in the cerebral ventricles will reverse this. An increase in THP has been noted in alcoholics. More notably, naloxone, an opiate antagonist, will block the self-stimulating effects of ETOH, suggesting that opiate receptors are involved. There may be a genetic defect in the peptidyl opiate system but more research is needed. Are alcoholics making their own opiates?

Another interesting finding of heuristic value is the fact that the alpha rhythm in the EEG, which is associated with relaxation and comfortableness, is reduced in alcoholics and their first-degree relatives. Alcohol increases alpha rhythm. Are alcoholics those people who basically cannot relax and have ser-endipitously discovered the solution?

Sociocultural
Certain subpopulations have been identified as a greater risk for alcoholism. Some of these and their characteristics are as follows:

Lower socioeconomic status (SES) males have higher rates of alcoholism but females have lower rates. Many years ago alcohol was inappropriately blamed for poverty and poverty for alcoholism. More alcoholics are seen in public hospitals and their populations are more predominately lower SES. Studies in some other countries, however, show a higher prevalence in upper classes. There are more DUIs and PIs in the lower SES, but this may be a bit skewed because of higher exposure to the police. Lower SES males are more apt to drink and drive. Basically, drinking problems are more concentrated in the lower half of the SES spectrum of males.

It is speculative as to why there is a higher prevalence in lower SES males, but observations have identified more entrap-ment in unrewarding, unenjoyable and even punitive job situations, higher unemployment, less hope for upward mobility, greater financial stress, lower ego strengths, less community support, higher impulsivity, fewer recreational opportunities, higher general stress levels, and poorer role models during developmental years.

Adolescents are showing an increasing prevalence of alcoholism in recent years although this may be levelling off. There is a higher use of drugs as well, so the state of altered consciousness becomes a sought after effect. The use of alcohol, including intoxication, by adolescents is identified as a rite of passage, identification with adults, rebellion against authority, peer initiation, evidence of superiority, successful competition (who can drink the most?), machismo, and narcissistic exhibitionism. These may be harmless enough and only transient but when combined with other problems, external and internal, the risks are greater. It is not at all unusual to see FHP males become clearly alcoholic in their teens, even early teens. Other commonalities of adolescence are an immature ego, emotional and narcissistic crises, pressures to succeed, identity struggles, unsatisfactory sexual experiences, and lability of affects. Getting drunk is not often peer dystonic. As long as alcoholic excursions are experimental and do not become a fixed and progressive pattern, there is usually no cause for alarm. If, however, drinking intensifies pathological acting out or progresses in severity then the person needs professional help. Professionals should study these youngsters in depth to attempt to tease out how much their psychopathology is cause and how much effect. Quite often these disturbed adolescents are from disturbed families and, in fact, this should be assumed to be so until proven otherwise.

Females have different drinking patterns and different causes than males. Their drinking begins later, is less daily, telescopes in progression more rapidly, and is less socially acceptable. They have more guilt feelings associated with it and have higher rates of suicidal attempts. In females there is a much higher prevalence of associated depression and a higher percentage of dual diagnoses, both physical and psychiatric. It causes even more family disruption, which in turn provides a feedback loop for further drinking. There is more solitary and secret drinking, and they are prone to emotional isolation. Sexual difficulties provoke more alienation by partners. The incidence of liver disease is higher. Stressors for women are higher: family tending is more demanding; societal demands for sex role stereotyping can be stifling; discrimination is still an unfortunate fact; sexual harrassment has not vanished; the general pattern of male attention to things and less to feelings has not changed, and less opportunity exists for recreational pursuits. A fairly high incidence of father-daughter incest has been found in their histories. It is not unusual to find a developmental history of a weak mother and a warm father, with whom the patient has identified with damaging feminine identity formation and self-worth. Arrests and job losses are fewer but damage to physical health and family is worse.

Tavern group. The custom of regular patronization of taverns probably traces back to English pubs which were the social, recreational and avocation centers for the working class. In the US today there seem to be two groups of tavern frequenters, the first being the working class, with a higher percentage of retired and disabled males, and the second being the young singles who use the setting for recreational and date-seeking purposes.

Skid row peoples are almost universally alcoholic. It is a way of life. Some of it, of course, is to escape the harshness and dreariness of their existence and to self-medicate for depression, but much of it sustains one of the few supports they have left – fellowship. It is unusual for a skid row person not to share a bottle. Death is the usual outcome, for obvious reasons.

Elderly. As stated earlier there is a U-shaped prevalence curve with age. The prevalence of alcoholism in the over 65 age group is high. There are three patterns: (a) Those who have always been alcoholic; (b) those who have always been mild problem drinkers but have a FHP history, and (c) those who have had neither of the above. It is generally thought this last group are almost always secondary alcoholics and that their drinking is stress produced. Corrective attention to their stressors in this last group is highly successful in reaching abstinence and they seldom need referral to AA. Common stressors for the elderly are a narrower circle of friends, bereavement, retirement, restricted economics, scattering of children and grandchildren, fewer hobbies, fewer support groups, health problems, more affect disregulation, and the existential matter of death. Their biology is also altered: there is much slower metabolism of alcohol (the customary two drinks at dinner may lead to clinical intoxication); decreased tolerance (for reasons not clearly understood); more toxicity, and more powerful clinical effects. Again, these people should not be seen as weak or treated with scorn, but identified as having symptoms of trouble and in need of help.

Male homosexuals who frequent gay bars as a part of their life style have higher levels of social and interpersonal anxiety and are at higher risk.

Behavioral

This is a concept which holds that drinking is a learned behavior and through repetition becomes a habit which is little under conscious control. This is much akin to the reward reinforcement paradigm. The theory here is that what has been learned can be unlearned by behavioral treatment techniques. More will be discussed further under treatment.

Psychodynamic

This point of view considers intrapsychic machinations which predispose to both increased risk and chronicity. These are interactional between the individual and his environment in maladaptive ways. These are often too complex and too subjective to lend themselves to statistical analysis yet are accepted as givens by clinicians in the field. Some have already been mentioned in the discussion of subpopulations and more will be discussed in the section on families.

Stress-producing internal dynamics can have multiple sources. These can be conceptualized as either primary, meaning pre-existing, or secondary, meaning resulting from alcohol. Most patients have both, and there is some overlapping. Many patients do not know why they drink, many will give excuses, often spurious, and some will reveal specific trouble areas.

Common areas of primary sources are: (a) unresolved conflicts, e.g., fixed hostile-dependency; (b) maturational arrests and deficits, e.g., failure at separation-individuation, poor role modeling for interpersonal relatedness or social skills; (c) subculturally derived prejudices, e.g., the paranoia of the lowest SES, and (d) issues stemming from dual diagnoses, e.g., the residual attention deficit disorder, or the intense abandonment anxiety of the borderline personality disorder. An entire list of examples is impractical. There is, incidentally, no such thing as the 'alcoholic personality', although this phrase is bandied about.

Secondary sources are universally found and become in themselves additive risk factors. Quite commonly found are guilt feelings, lowered self-esteem, built up anger because of frustrated omnipotent strivings, thwarted demands for nurturance and control over their worlds, and intensified dependency. Losses of spouses, support systems, jobs and brushes with the law are common, leading to further humiliation and resentment. Depression is a frequent result.

Commonly seen in alcoholics as both primary and secondary dynamics are denial (not only of the alcoholism but effects as well), a chronic sense of inadequacy (usually defended by masked grandiosity and a compulsive drive for mastery), cumulative suppressed and repressed anger, excessive dependency, and chronic guilt feelings (which are not only perpetual internal torment but provocative of hypersensitivity to criticism).

17

These dynamic issues can be seen as not fixed or static but as operating in a dynamic feedback continuum between the patient, his family and his associates.

Intrapsychic factors leading to progression are conditioned euphoria, conditioned relief of anxiety and depression, denial of a downward spiral of social, psychological and environmental supports, suppression and repression of guilt feelings, loss of self-esteem and loss of fancied omnipotence. We do not know how much progression provokes more denial or denial contributes to further progression, although both exist, but denial is a hallmark characteristic of the disease. The quantity of these factors varies in each individual and is difficult to measure. They do interrelate with other risk factors.

Factors influencing these stem from a number of sources: hereditary constitution; traumata; inner conflicts; failures in development; identifications; DSM-III-R disorders; physical disease, and organic brain damage.

A healthy person has not only the capacities to love and to work, but also to be comfortably and productively involved in the world. Impairments in ego strength are usually persistent, although there is usually the innate capacity for growth. Assisting the person in realization of some of this potential for growth is one of the responsibilities and pleasures of psychotherapy.

Ego Strength

Successful coping with life, management of drives and needs, and dealing with affects are regulated by ego strengths. It entails how we all perceive, process and respond to our outer and inner worlds. It involves accuracy of perception, the ability to weigh meaning and significance, reality testing, prediction of outcome of intended speech and action, judgement and ability to plan. It also involves intelligence, coping skills, sense of humor, resiliency, ability to learn from experience, flexibility, and the capacity to love and share. It also involves such things as psychological mindedness, ability to tolerate stress and frustration, decision making, affect modulation, integrity, honesty, freedom from stereotypes and repetition compulsions, accuracy of self-perception, adequacy of self-esteem, ability to grieve losses, optimism, adequacy of social skills, relationships with authority, ability to find pleasures, levels of inner tension, and creativity. This is not a complete list nor meant to serve as a precise definition, but to be useful for appraisal purposes. None of these features are to be seen as absolutes but as characteristics which are of varying quantity and quality and which influence the management of stress and the quality of life.

Stress

Stress can be seen as originating externally or internally. Not infrequently these are interactional and mutually contributory. Examples of internal stress have been briefly outlined in the section on dynamics. External stressors are too numerous to mention. Death of a spouse, death of a child, unemployment, divorce, poverty, homelessness, chronic incapacitating illness are examples of severe stress. A great many alcoholics blame stress as the 'cause' of their drinking, and while it may well be a factor it is much more likely that the etiology is based more on other factors, especially deficits in ego strength and heredity. Nonetheless, stress cannot be ignored in the assessment of the alcoholic and efforts in therapy to reduce stress whenever possible are worthwhile. It is particularly important to address those stressors which are self-induced, either neurotically or as a result of drinking. One stress which is both external and internal is aging. Freud stated in 'Civilization and Its Discontents', 'Life as we find it is too hard for us: it entails too much pain, too many disappointments, impossible tasks. We cannot do without palliative remedies. There are perhaps three of these means: powerful diversion of interests, substitute gratifications which lessen it, and intoxication which makes us insensitive to it.' Seeking relief from tension is quite probably a homeostatic phenomenon.

Thus we see no single risk factor as the cause of alcoholism. It is a very complex biopsychosocial disease. Our best approach in understanding and treatment is detailed investigation of each particular individual with respect to their multiple risk factors. Multidisciplinary remedial approaches to reversible risk factors are the only intelligent systems of rehabilitation and should be combined with AA. No in-patient alcohol rehabilitation center can adequately address all of these issues given their time constraints and impracticalities.

5 Taking a History

In addition to a standard psychiatric history and survey of risk factors, a bit more information is needed in assessing the severity, duration, damages, previous treatment efforts and motivation for change in these individuals. The following areas give a useful outline.

There are quantitative and qualitative differences in *drinking patterns.* Items to investigate are: amount consumed; types of beverage; diurnal pattern; daily drinking or sprees or both; when drinking starts during the day; solitary or with others and where; 'eye openers'; periods of abstinence; what degree of progression over what period of time; age when drinking started; age when drinking became out of control, and duration of out of control periods.

The *consequences* of drinking need to be inquired into, not only with the patient but also with significant others, including Employee Assistance Personnel, due to typical untruthfulness, minimization and denial. A useful question is, 'What has happened to you and your world since your drinking has been out of control?' One can look into repetitive types of pathological behavior during intoxication, history of blackouts, DTs, memory loss, arrests for DIU or PI, seizures, diminished ability to concentrate, diminished energy level, sex drive changes, liver, pancreatic, gastric, or neurological disease, tremors, injuries, and hangovers. Personal areas to look into are: fighting; marital problems; family problems; deterioration in peer groups; poorer job performance; job warnings; job losses; comments by people other than family; loss of self-esteem; problems with personal finances; loss of physical health; depression; loss of ambition; abandonment of hobbies and interests.

What *previous treatment* for both detoxification and rehabilitation has the person had? One seeks details of where, when, duration, follow-up and aftercare, attendance at AA, attitudes toward AA, self-participation in AA, relationship with sponsor, duration of AA attendance, use of token clubs and other AA activities. What made the person slip, if they know?

Problems in *interpersonal relationships* can contribute to and result from alcoholism. Is the spouse and/or family an enabler? What has the drinking done to peer groups, social invitations and personal friendships and how has the alcoholic reacted to these? What has happened to general support systems, e.g., church, hobbies, special interest groups, reading, etc.? Has there been deterioration in personality functioning? What has happened to the quality of life since drinking became out of control? How does the person deal with the urge to and invitations to drink?

Personality trait disturbances are frequent in alcoholism, sometimes pre-existing and assisting in contributing to risk factors and sometimes being a result of drinking and then giving feedback to both. Assessment of these by observation, further interviews, psychological tests and history from family members is useful in evaluating pre-existing traits and alcohol-produced or -exaggerated traits over time.

As a part of the examination of the problem drinker, it is also important to look *inside* the person. What feelings and affects has the person repressed or lacks, and which have deteriorated with abuse? What does alcohol 'do' for the person? Does the person admit to being an alcoholic? How seriously do they admit it? Does the person admit to powerlessness over drinking? What are their motivations for the goal of abstinence? What inner conflict areas exist and how does the person deal with them?

The assessment of the drinker is not complete without a *family history* of alcoholism and other psychopathology. Alcoholism patterns in family members should be identified for presence, severity, duration, consequences and outcome. The same assessment should be done for family personality traits, parental patterns of child rearing and relationships, existing DSM-III-R Axes I or II disorders, and current quantity and quality of familial interpersonal relationships. These should be done to assess heredity, support systems, pathological identifications, areas of conflict, traumata, and current conflicts in relationships.

A search for possible *DSM-III-R Axes I and/or II disorders* should be done in the patient. The incidence of these is quite high, quite possibly 60% as a conservative estimate. If present these need further evaluation as to date of onset, family history, progression, details of illness, details of previous treatment, effects upon and effects from drinking. Some are pre-existing and co-existing as dual diagnoses. Some are primary and some are secondary diseases, although alcoholism is always to be seen as a primary disease unto itself. Equal attention to these multiple disorders is essential to more favorable outcomes in treatment.

There is a clear relationship between pathological reality testing, stereotyped behavior and unstable attitudes, thinking and behaviors and a reduction in the quality of life and the quality and quantity of supports.

People do affect others for better or worse. When inappropriate, unrealistic, thoughtless or hostile behavior or remarks are made by the patient then *environmental responses* tend to be negative. This results in frustration and disappointment with resulting anger, helplessness, dysphoria and perplexity. Depending on the importance and meaning of the negative environmental response and the alcoholic's level of frustration tolerance their defenses may not be adequate, leading to further maladaptation, further jousting with the environment and more dysphoria. Repetition of the same themes over time not only provokes immediate negative environmental responses but is very apt, as well, to lead to subsequent rejection, withdrawal, retaliation or abandonment. Alcoholic behavior itself is provocative enough, but when compounded by rejection the combination is synergistic.

Changes in personality and life style are equally as important in the recovery process as are direct efforts to maintain abstinence, since all of these influence relapse. Recovery is never just abstinence alone. If the person does not change psychic factors which are changeable, they become what is known in the field of alcoholism as a 'dry drunk', someone who is sober but is the same person with the same problems, same attitudes and often the same interpersonal behavior, and is at much greater risk for relapse as well as deterioration of supports. AA calls this 'stinking thinking'.

6 Metabolism

Alcohol is one of the few substances absorbed through the gastric mucosa as well as the intestines, partially accounting for its rapidity of effects.

85% of alcohol is metabolized in the liver by two pathways, 15% is eliminated unchanged in the breath, urine and sweat. In the liver 80% is oxidized by the dehydrogenase systems and 20% by the microsomal ethanol-oxidizing systems (MEOSs).

The dehydrogenase system is as follows: alcohol + alcohol dehydrogenase (ADH) and the coenzyme nicotinamide adenine dinucleotide (NAD) $\rightarrow$ acetaldehyde (AcH). AcH + AcH dehydrogenase and coenzyme A $\rightarrow$ acetate and H_2O. Acetate + amino acids, via citric acid cycle $\rightarrow$ CO_2, O_2, H, ketone bodies, fatty acids and steroid synthesis. This process takes place in the liver mitochondria. Individual livers show two groups of ADH, normal and atypical, and there are at least eight fractions of ADH. Genetic differences exist. Not all the pathways of AcH metabolism are known. Offspring of alcoholics show higher levels of AcH than non-alcoholics with test doses of ETOH, even prior to the onset of alcoholism. There are differences in this system in different ethnic groups – approximately 90% of orientals have quite high AcH levels with alcohol. There are other pathways for Ach metabolism, not all of them known, and these may have some qualitative importance.

The MEOS consists of microsomal enzymes which oxidize alcohol, but the part they play in metabolism is not yet well understood. It is known that chronic alcohol use produces a proliferation of these. Since these also oxidize other substances, such as anesthetic agents, this may partly explain why chronic alcoholics are more resistive to anesthetics.

Alcoholic beverages contain other alcohols that ethyl, and the higher the alcohol in molecular weight the more affinity there is for these enzyme systems. Alcohol congeners also contain alcohols, all of which have a high affinity for ADH. There is one therapeutic use for ETOH and that is for emergency use after the ingestion of methyl alcohol or of ethyl glycol (antifreeze). These have lower molecular weights than ETOH and thus can be slowed down in their metabolism and toxic effects since ETOH successfully competes for metabolism with them.

Blood alcohol levels begin to fall about 2 h after ingestion ceases and, unless there is significant liver disease or the subject is elderly, are usually down to zero in 12–24 h.

7 Acetaldehyde

AcH is important enough to warrant discussion in a separate section. Its effects are greater than ETOH alone.

It has multiple metabolic pathways and effects. It structurally resembles the hallucinogens (perhaps a factor in alcoholic hallucinations). It has neuropharmacologic and biologic reactions of its own. Its effects parallel those seen with *d*-amphetamine. It is 35 times more potent in producing intoxication in mice. It is a general metabolic stimulant. It is quite volatile and therefore hard to study. There are higher concentrations of it in alcoholics.

In the nervous system it acts first as a stimulant and then as a depressant. Brain AcH levels are equal to or greater than blood alcohol levels (BALs). There is a higher concentration in the cerebellum. It is what causes 'hangover' effects of headache, nausea, and jitteriness. It is potentiated by cocaine. It lowers brain norepinephrine and serotonin. It reacts with dopamine to produce the isoquinolines.

Other effects are stimulation of CHO metabolism to produce hyperglycemia (hypoglycemia in the malnourished) and interference with gluconeogenesis. It decreases urinary 5-hydroxyindoleacetic acid, vanillyl mandelic acid and 3-methoxy-4-hydroxyphenylglycol (related to production of frequent depression?). It mobilizes free fatty acids and triglycerides. It changes ketone metabolism. It releases peripheral catecholamines and this effect lasts longer than detoxification, resulting in hypertension. It gives a biphasic reaction in the heart, at first giving a transient increase and then a second and more lasting decrease in rate and contractility.

8 Laboratory Findings

There are no pathognomonic laboratory markers of alcoholism, with the exception of the BAL in certain circumstances. A BAL of over 100 in a routine examination or over 150 without any clinical signs of intoxication is indicative of alcoholism. BAL is underutilized and could well be routine in physical workups. The clinical history is more reliable than the laboratory in the diagnosis of alcoholism, although computer quadratic discriminant analysis, which is not readily available clinically, of 24 commonly ordered tests has identified 100% of non-alcoholics and 98% of alcoholics. Laboratory abnormalities are nonetheless useful for screening purposes, evaluation of severity of tissue pathology and monitoring recovery and abstinence.

A macrocytic anemia is not uncommon with heavy drinking, due to direct toxicity and decreased folate and B_{12}. A mean corpuscular volume (MCV) of over 96 (which may last for a month after cessation), macrocytosis, hemoglobin less than 14 g in males and less than 12.5 g in females are indicative of marrow suppression. Pancytopenia can be found. A leukocytosis suggests infection.

Blood chemistry will sometimes find abnormalities. The most sensitive is the GGT, which is abnormal above 30–35 units/l. 70% of heavy drinkers will have an elevated GGT. It appears before other liver enzymes become abnormal. Other conditions such as diabetes, obesity, pregnancy, various drugs and hepatitis can also elevate this, and 15% of normal drinkers have been found to have abnormal GGT levels.

Other abnormalities to be alert to, but occurring with lesser frequency are as follows. There are increases in aspartate aminotransferase (AST or SGOT), alanine aminotransferase (ALT or SGPT), creatinine phosphokinase (CPK), alkaline phosphatase (ALP), lactic dehydrogenase (LDH), uric acid, glucose, phosphorus, chlorides, bilirubin, cholesterol, and triglycerides. High density lipoproteins are increased. Serum IgA is increased in those with liver disease. Plasma osmolality and serum lactate are increased during intoxication and as long as ETOH is being metabolized. Elevations in serum lactate may be quite helpful in identifying drunk drivers. There are decreases in total protein, albumin, calcium, serum iron, CO_2, B_{12} and folate.

Attempts to use certain laboratory profiles, such as GGT, MCV, AST, and ALP in screening and monitoring are under further study.

The CT scan of the brain will demonstrate ventricular enlargement in a higher percentage of cases than expected.

9 General Physiology

Many different biological processes are affected by alcohol. Specific organ pathology will be discussed under a separate section below.

Alcohol goes to the hydrophobic regions of cell membranes. It goes across membranes by simple diffusion. It is not absorbed through the skin. Its plasma/tissue concentration is directly proportional to the H_2O content.

Every aspect of CHO metabolism is affected. It influences the output of insulin and decreases gluconeogenesis. There are changes in ketone metabolism as mentioned in the section on metabolism. The uric acid cycle is decreased. Increased hepatic NAD/NADH ratio gives increased lactate which gives hyperuricemia, one of the frequently found laboratory markers.

There is decreased absorption of amino acids and decreased transamination and deamination of amino acids.

There is an increased rate of O_2 consumption leading to tissue O_2 deficiency, which affects the liver in chronic alcoholics. As previously noted, it increases the alpha rhythm in the EEG. The diuretic response occurs only when the BAL is rising. This gives a thirst, which is sometimes mistaken for dehydration. There is a 3- to 10-fold increase in urine flow, but without any increase in electrolyte excretion. Chronic alcoholics have an increase in total body H_2O, both in plasma and in cells, including the brain. Intravenous fluids are contraindicated for detoxification, unless the subject is truly dehydrated clinically from malnutrition.

Congeners increase the degree and duration of EEG changes and increase the depressant effects.

Intoxication produces earlier onset of sleep but decreased rapid eye movement (REM) time.

There are many nonpharmacologic factors which influence the rapidity, degree and effects of intoxication such as expectancy, previous experience, the setting, sought after ego syntonic effects, and levels of dysphoria.

10 Tolerance and Dependence

While there are individual differences in the degree and duration of tolerance, it generally develops linearly with frequency, amount and duration of drinking. It begins to develop after the first drink, ultimately reaches a plateau with continued drinking, and in many subjects will gradually decline (known as 'reverse tolerance') to quite low levels after many, many years.

It is primarily a tissue adaptation although there is a slight increase in the MEOS. Psychosocial factors also influence tolerance to some degree.

Tolerance can reach as high as a BAL of 0.30 mg% or even higher without demonstrable motor impairment in those who have developed an unusually high tolerance. A BAL of more than 0.15 mg% in anyone without clinical signs of intoxication is pathognomonic for alcoholism.

There is a cross-tolerance to all other sedating agents, meaning that it takes equally larger amounts of sedatives and anesthetics to be effective. Any drug with sedating properties will be involved in this effect of x-tolerance. This is why, for example, there is a considerable percent of fatality in heroin and other opioid addicts who also use alcohol – the tolerance to each brings blood levels to dangerously high levels and that, plus additive factors, becomes lethal. There is x-tolerance also to benzodiazepines and tetrahydrocannabinol.

Tolerance is generally reversible although in some people it remains high even after protracted abstinence.

Dependence is of two types, physical and psychological. The physical is acquired rapidly if the intake is over 3 oz of absolute alcohol per day. The physical is more reversible than the psychological. The psychological consists of the craving, which is due to both the physical dependence and to psychological ego-syntonic euphorigenic and palliative effects.

II Organ Pathology

Nervous System

In addition to the acute effects on the nervous system during intoxication and during withdrawal (described elsewhere) the nervous system is injured sooner, more frequently and more seriously than any other organ system in alcoholism. The brain is damaged sooner than the liver in chronic alcoholics.

Brain damage is due to cellular necrosis and is related to the duration and degree of drinking. It is not due to vitamin deficiency, except for the Wernicke-Korsakoff syndrome. Even moderate drinking, if persistent, has been demonstrated to give decreased cognitive performance, recent memory, problem solving, abstraction and monitoring simultaneous information from multiple sources. 35–50% of hospitalized alcoholics in alcohol treatment programs show some deficits on neuropsychological testing, most of which can be reversed in time, but which may last up to a year or more following abstinence. (This is important to evaluate during treatment.) 40–70% of chronic alcoholics show increased size of brain ventricles and cortical atrophy on CT scan. All chronic alcoholics, even those in their 20s, show some cerebral atrophy, (more frontal in the young), and even heavy social drinkers may show atrophy. The hippocampus and cerebellum are more vulnerable. This atrophy will improve somewhat after 1–3 years of abstinence. Continued abuse also results in behavioral change, some of which is organically based, e.g., inability to learn new information.

Organic mental disorders due to alcohol are listed in DSM-III-R as: (1) alcohol intoxication; (2) alcoholic idiosyncratic intoxication; (3) uncomplicated alcohol withdrawal;

(4) alcohol withdrawal delirium; (5) alcohol hallucinosis; (6) alcohol amnestic disorder, and (7) dementia associated with alcoholism. The reader is referred to these. The Wernicke-Korsakoff encephalopathy (included in dementia) is a progressive degenerative disease, especially in the periventricular area of the brain, associated with a triad of dementia, ataxia and ocular abnormalities. As much as 3 % of alcoholics in charity hospitals have this. It occurs after only many years of heavy drinking, usually appearing when the alcoholics are in their 50s. Confabulation is frequently associated with the dementia. The dementia improves in only 15 %. The ocular abnormalities are nystagmus, abducens palsy and palsy of conjugate gaze. The gait disturbance is permanent in 60 % of cases. There is a 20 % mortality, not from the disorder per se but from other causes. Only 20 % recover. It is caused by thiamine deficiency, which causes tissue necrosis. Thiamine in large doses parentally is the treatment.

Peripheral neuritis has an insidious onset, is bilateral, and involves both motor and sensory components. Paresthesias, motor weakness, muscle atrophy and decreased sensation of all types are found. Conduction velocities are decreased, the EMG shows degeneration and there is polyneuropathy on biopsy. It can show in chronic alcoholics of at least 10 years duration and is due to nutritional and thiamine deficiency. Treatment is with a high calorie diet and large doses of B vitamins.

Respiration

The respiratory center is depressed during rebound leading to lowered O_2 and to respiratory alkalosis. The latter results in a shift in magnesium, important in withdrawal tremors, DT and withdrawal seizures. More will be discussed under the section on detoxification.

Clearing mechanisms of the respiratory tree are impaired due to suppression of ciliary activities by alcohol. This is one factor in the higher incidence of pulmonary infections.

Alcoholics smoke tobacco more than twice as heavily as the non-alcoholic adult population, another factor in lowering resistance since nicotine sharply reduces ciliary action. Chronic bronchitis is common.

Alcohol interfers with the cough reflex and phagocytosis thus further impairing resistance.

Bronchitis, pneumonia, lung abscess, tuberculosis, bronchiectasis and pleural effusion are not uncommon.

Cardiovascular

Hypertension is common. This may persist for a month or two following abstinence. It should be noted that ETOH will aggravate hypertension from other causes. Antihypertensive medication should be very cautiously prescribed in mild hypertension because many such agents are depressionogenic and add a risk factor for alcohol relapse. Hypertension is common in those who have more than two drinks per day. The cardiovascular effects of ETOH are dose-dependent.

Increased catecholamines, over hydration, and electrolyte changes have a vasodilatory effect on blood vessels, especially capillaries in the skin, but a vasoconstrictive effect in muscles.

Cardiac impairment can be to varying degrees, the severest being in alcoholic cardiomyopathy. Triglyceride content in the myocardium is increased; hyponatremia promotes arrhythmias; myocardial protein synthesis is lowered; there is less coronary flow; there is less energy production; muscle fibers are damaged; there is less contractility, and there is lowered ejection fraction and functional reserve. ECG changes are nonspecific and consist of extrasystoles, atrial fibrillation and bundle branch block. Cardiac work is increased. There is no connection per se to the production or course of coronary artery pathology, but those with coronary disease should not drink because of the myocardial effects of ETOH. There is hypertrophy, degeneration of muscle fibers, fibrosis and fibroblastosis. Muscle fibers show hyalination, edema, vacuolization and granularity. Symptoms of alcoholic cardiomyopathy are shortness of breath, dependent edema, decreased exercise tolerance, persistent tachycardia, ischemic chest pain, anorexia, abnormal sweating on exertion, and nocturnal leg cramps. The heart shows considerable enlargement. Alcoholic pericardiopathy characterized by pericardial effusion, increased circulation time, and ECG changes consistent with pericarditis is seen in beer drinkers and is due to the cobalt in beer.

While not as common as other cardiovascular complications stroke can occur as a result of alcoholism, sometimes independent of hypertension. These are usually hemorrhagic rather then embolic.

Gastrointestinal

There is a definite increase in the prevalance of esophageal cancer in alcoholics. This is not, however, associated with those who drink only wine or beer. There is also decreased peristalsis, but this is usually asymptomatic. Acute and chronic gastritis, with heme-positive stools, is due to two factors. Alcohol, even given parenterally, increases the secretion of HCl (this gradually diminishes in chronic alcoholics and disappears after 6 months for unknown reasons). There is acute mucosal injury with hyperemia, erosion and bleeding, and with ulcerations, if severe. Alcohol breaks down the gastric mucosal barrier and also alters the lipid-protein layer of the surface resulting in acid penetration of the cellular junctions. There is very little evidence that ETOH produces peptic ulcer disease but it will aggravate it, if pre-existing.

There are tissue changes in the wall of the small intestine (somewhat similar to the cellular damage seen in the liver) consisting of focal cellular degeneration and protoplasmic proliferation. These changes result in malabsorption of CHO, amino acids, and vitamins B, B_{12} and E. There are also alterations in peristalsis.

Liver

There are three types of liver disease in alcoholism: fatty liver, acute hepatitis, and cirrhosis. There is some suggestion that there can be a progression of these in the order just named. All involve steatosis.

Pathogenesis has multiple causes. Fat is the main fuel for the liver but ETOH is more preferred thus fatty acids, both dietary and endogenously produced, accumulate in the liver. ETOH produces cellular membrane changes. There is lowered O_2 tension (from multiple causes) leading to pericentral hypoxia resulting in cellular damage and release of enzymes. (There is a 30–60% decrease in the rate of O_2 consumption.) There is a decrease in fatty acid oxidation and an increase in lipid synthesis and peroxidation. Microsomes are activated. Enzymes are increased. There is lowered liver blood flow. Increased AcH is hepatotoxic. Secretion of albumin and glycoproteins are inhibited with resultant hepatocellular retention. Mitochondria become swollen and distorted in shape. There is a decreased NAD/NADH ratio. Malnutrition and heredity are not factors.

Fatty Liver

Biopsy of the liver in 100 problem drinkers showed that 65% had fatty liver disease. It can occur even in social drinkers where inebriation has not been present. The cells show enlargement, vacuolar dilatation, proliferation of endoplasmic reticulum, cytoplasmic degeneration with focal vacuoles, swollen and distorted mitochondria. There may be fatty cysts. A steady intake of 100–170 g/day is sufficient to produce a fatty liver. A high fat and low protein diet may contribute.

The liver is enlarged, smooth and non-tender. There are seldom clinical symptoms although in more severe cases anorexia, anergia, abdominal pain, nausea, vomiting and jaundice can occur. It usually reverses with abstinence. It is only rarely fatal and then due to an obstructive syndrome. Increased GGT, other liver enzymes, bilirubin, uric acid and glycosylated hemoglobin are often found. Treatment is abstinence and a high protein, low fat diet.

Alcoholic Hepatitis

This probably differs from fatty liver more quantitatively than qualitatively. There is an enlarged and tender liver. Cellular necrosis and inflammation are added to fatty liver. There is intracytoplasmic inclusion of hyaline. Mallory bodies, consisting of a mix of strands, granules and aggragates, often surrounded by polymorphonuclear leukocytes are found.

Symptoms are anorexia, nausea, fever, abdominal pain, and a tender and enlarged liver. It has a more serious prognosis than fatty liver and only 62% have a 5-year survival after the onset of the disease. It can go to renal failure.

In addition to the laboratory findings listed above for fatty liver there is leukocytosis and a decreased prothrombin. The SGOT is higher than the SGPT. An unremitting prothrombin has a grave prognosis. Diagnosis is confirmed by biopsy. Treatment is a high protein, low fat diet. Propanolol and calcium channel blockers may reduce hypoxic damage. Propylthiouricil and colchicine have promise. Prednisolone is generally contraindicated.

Alcoholic Cirrhosis

There are diffuse fibrous bands in portal and central zones with disruption of lobular architecture, inflammation, varying amounts of necrosis, cholestasis, bile duct proliferation and siderosis. Initially the liver is enlarged but as the disease progresses it decreases in size, eventually to less than premorbid size. The liver is nodular and progresses from micro- to macronodular. The disorder is twice as frequent in males and occurs only after many years (approximately 24) of heavy drinking. The average age of onset is 50 and the average age of death is between 55 and 60. There is a correlation with the amount and duration of alcohol and cirrhosis.

Approximately 160 g/day for 6–10 years gives an 8% incidence, after 11–15 years a 21% incidence, more than 180 g/day for more than 15 years a 51% incidence. Initially the symptoms are weight loss, weakness and anorexia. As it progresses there is jaundice. Tertiary symptoms are fever, ascites, esophageal and gastric varices, peripheral edema, spider nevi, pulmonary edema, Dupuytren's contracture, clubbing, testicular atrophy, decreased body hair with female distribution, gynecomastia, splenic enlargement and hepatic encephalopathy. The encephalopathy progresses from precoma to coma to death and is accompanied by asterixis and a slowing of the EEG to 4 or less. Scans show areas of decreased uptake. Bilirubin can become quite high. A megaloblastic anemia from bone marrow depression, decreased folic acid and B_{12}, and increased activity of the spleen is common. Renal hemodynamics are lowered leading to decreased blood flow and oliguria. A lower K^+ is found.

Treatment is abstinence, limiting dietary protein, neomycin to decrease proteolytic and urea splitting enzymes in the gut, sodium restriction, sorbital which acidifies the stool thus promoting ammonia excretion, supplemental K^+, and spironolactone up to 400 mg/day. The anemia should be addressed. Steroids are to be avoided as they increase fatality. Fiberoptic endoscopy procedures and vasopressin infusions can be used for bleeding varices. Levodopa can be used for encephalopathy. One should be very cautious with sedatives and tranquilizers since these are metabolized in the liver and quite high plasma levels of these drugs are likely to occur. Surgical shunting of the portal system has a high mortality. For those maintaining abstinence for a year beyond initial diagnosis and treatment, the survival rate is 86%. Oliguria and azotemia have a grave prognosis.

Pancreas

30–40% of acute pancreatitis is from alcohol. Both acute and chronic pancreatitis of a nonspecific type is not rare in alcoholics. It is usually in males in their 4th decade.

It usually has a fairly acute onset. Symptoms are severe sharp epigastric pain with radiation through to the back, nausea, vomiting, tachycardia, and some temperature elevation. Psychotic delirium can infrequently occur.

Serum amylase is usually greater than 500 Somogyi units, although it is normal in 10–20%. Leukocytosis, increased lipase, increased blood sugar and decreased calcium are common laboratory findings. X-rays often show pancreatic calcification, sentinal loops of the ileus, left-sided pleural effusion and basal pulmonary atelectasis. Ultrasonography may distinguish the type of pancreatic enlargement. Large amounts of fluid can be lost in the retroperitoneal space.

A chronic course can sometimes occur. Recurrences with continued drinking are common. Complications are diabetes mellitus, cholestasis, pancreatic ascites and pseudocysts. 90% survive.

Treatment is with analgesics, such as pentazocine or phenazocine, which have a minimal effect on the sphincter of Oddi-pentazocine or phenazocine, nasogastric suction and intravenous fluids.

Hematologic

Different abnormalities in hematology occur in alcoholism. Anemias can be from blood loss, iron deficiency, folic acid or B_{12} deficiency, and bone marrow depression.

Alcohol itself has a toxic depressive effect on bone marrow. There is a pancytopenia. This can occur even in well-nourished alcoholics. The depression produces a decrease in production of all types of blood cells and clotting factors. There is vacuolization of marrow precursor cells. Alcoholism is the most common cause of thrombocytopenia in the US.

Both folic acid and B_{12}, which are reduced in alcoholics, are essential in the synthesis of DNA precursors and these are in turn essential for granulocytes, megakaryocytes and platelets.

Folate deficiency from alcohol itself, poorer intestinal absorption and poor diet contributes to the megaloblastic anemia. This is less in beer drinkers since beer contains folate.

Abnormal accumulations of iron granules in red blood cells and marrow precursors, deposited in the mitochondria surrounding the nucleus, known as ring siderosis, are common. Serum iron levels may be increased but fall during detoxification indicating increased use of iron by the bone marrow. There is a decrease in pyridoxine phosphate, an enzyme in Fe metabolism.

These effects last only a few days to a week after cessation of drinking. There is a rebound thrombocytosis and a rebound leukocytosis.

Alcohol also reduces phytohemagglutin and antigen-induced lymphocyte transformation. It also impairs lymphocyte transport. These factors impair the immune response to infection.

MCV is often elevated, one of the laboratory markers for alcoholism. Hematocrit is often normal but falls after several days of sobriety due to rehydration.

If there is cirrhosis of the liver there is a hemolytic anemia and lowered vitamin K with resultant decreased coagulation and fibrinolysis.

ETOH also diminishes the production of thymus-derived lymphocytes, thus further lowering immune defenses.

Endocrine

The hypothalamic-pituitary-adrenal axis activity is increased for 2–4 weeks after cessation of drinking. Increased plasma cortisol levels and an abnormal dexamethasone suppression test are commonly found, and should not be confused with an endogenous depression.

There is an increase in norepinephrine turnover and enhanced central nervous system (CNS) adrenergic receptor binding in the brain. Other CNS compounds involved in withdrawal are prolactin, thyrotropin-releasing hormone, vasopressin, cyclic adenosine monophosphate and delta sleep-inducing peptides. Vasopressin reduction leads to diuresis. Triiodothyronine and thyroxine levels are decreased.

Prostaglandins, leukotrienes and thromboxanes are decreased resulting in less smooth muscle contraction, increased capillary permeability, decreased platelet aggregation and dis-aggregation, bronchoconstriction, cardiac dysfunction and de-creased polymorphonuclear leukocyte accumulation at sites of infection. Prostaglandins also protect against alcoholic fatty liver and protect the gastric mucosa.

There is hypogonadism, testicular atrophy and lowered testosterone in the male in chronic alcoholics. Impotence (also caused by alcoholic neuropathy of the pelvic nerves), decreased sperm count and decreased libido are common in many chronic alcoholics. There is also a higher conversion of androgen to estrogen, further contributing to sexual problems and also pro-ducing gynecomastia and feminine hair distribution. Testoster-one levels may never return to normal with abstinence so the damage may be permanent. Menstrual disorders, decreased vaginal blood flow and a higher incidence of breast and thyroid cancer are seen in women.

Muscle

Muscle pathology stems from both the toxic effects of alcohol on muscle fibers and the effects of polyneuropathy. ETOH is a toxin for striated muscle. Polyneuropathy, both from toxic and nutritional sources, is characterized by demyeliniza-tion and neuronal denervation. The onset is usually insidious. Weakness, decreased sensation and diminished reflexes are found. The EMG shows denervation, conduction velocities are reduced and biopsy shows polyneuropathy. It occurs usually only after extensive drinking for at least 10 years. It can be acute with necrosis and myoglobinuria but this is rare. More commonly there is progressive weakness, atrophy and sensory changes. Treatment is a high calorie diet, B vitamins, especially thiamine, and when indicated potassium and magnesium.

12 Intoxication

The effects of intoxication parallel the ascending or descending blood alcohol levels to some extent, with ego syntonic and stimulating effects associated with ascending and dystonic and sedative effects with descending levels. A generalization, however, is that the degree of intoxication parallels the peak BAL. The following scale is only approximate:

0.020–0.099 mg%	= impaired coordination, euphoria
0.100–0.199 mg%	= ataxia, impaired cognition, poor judgment, labile mood
0.200–0.299 mg%	= marked ataxia, slurred speech, poor judgment
0.300–0.399 mg%	= stage-I anesthesia, memory lapse, labile mood
0.440+ mg%	= respiratory failure, coma, death

BALs and stages of clinical intoxication do not, however, have an exact linear relationship. There are large individual differences. High levels of tolerance, however, will influence these BALs and their effects. It is possible for an alcoholic with considerable tolerance to have a BAL of 0.150 mg% and not be clinically intoxicated. 1 oz of whiskey = 1 glass of wine = 12 oz beer = 0.025 mg% BAL.

Intoxication produces psychic effects of loquaciousness, mood changes, disinhibition, impaired discrimination and judgment, inappropriate expressions of affects and repressed impulses, anxiety, euphoria, dysphoria. It becomes anxiolytic for the most part, and this may be one of the factors responsible for disinhibition. Motor effects are slowed reflexes and reaction times, impaired coordination, ataxia, slurred speech, nystagmus, body sway.

The severity of intoxication depends on the rapidity of intake and the ascent of the BAL, the peak level, tolerance and the presence of other drugs. There is a discordance between subjective and objective appraisal of levels of intoxication. Alcoholics have a wider discrepancy in this appraisal than non-alcoholics. FHP alcoholics have less subjective intoxication, less body sway and less impairment on trails making tests. An empty stomach and less body weight increases the rapidity of the rise in the BAL with comparable amounts of ETOH. There are no basic differences between alcoholics and non-alcoholics on the time to peak BAL, its magnitude or rate of decline, except in the elderly. The elderly have less body mass, less mitochondrial activity, more toxicity and slower metabolism. Females have a more rapidly ascending BAL and have 35–45% higher peak BALs than males, partly due to more rapid absorption. Oral contraceptives inhibit metabolism with resulting higher peaks and slower decreases in BAL.

The alcohol 'idiosyncratic intoxication syndrome' is outlined in DSM-III-R and will not be repeated here. It is highly apt to be recurrent. It is not rare to see violence associated with this. It can be confused with temporal lobe epilepsy or drug intoxication, especially phencyclidine. Treatment should be the same as for any other psychosis. Such subjects should be appropriately cautioned and treated. Patients with this syndrome may have abnormal EEGs to begin with, frontal and temporal lobe spikes, bursts of high voltage slow 2–6/s waves or a mixture of spike and slow wave bursts.

Intoxication may precipitate seizures in an epileptic. These are not, however, withdrawal seizures. Thermal regulation is sometimes disturbed and there is a low grade fever.

Magnesium is lowered due to decreased intake, malabsoprtion, excess renal loss, and respiratory alkalosis. Potassium is shifted into cells. Sodium is retained.

Thiamine deficiency is quite common. Generally, however, there is no deficiency in the other vitamins, unless there is definite malnutrition.

Catecholamine release from tissues, not the adrenals, gives an increase in pulse and blood pressure, often lasting 1–4 weeks after detoxification.

Rebound insomnia and increased REM on the EEG may last 1–4 weeks after cessation of drinking.

Effects on neurotransmitters have been mentioned. Hyperlipidemia is frequent as a result of metabolism.

13 Indications for Hospitalization

While there have been some reports stating that inpatient treatment of alcoholics is no better than outpatient, these have not been studied scientifically rigorously and do not fit the experience of experts in the field. While a great many can be treated as outpatients, the decision to hospitalize should be individualized and based on clinical judgment of the many variables. The following are guidelines for hospitalization:

1   Moderately severe to severe withdrawal symptoms
2   Failure of outpatient treatment
3   Concurrent physical disease or injury sufficient to need daily medical and nursing attention
4   History of DTs or withdrawal seizures in the past
5   Inadequate support systems
6   Dual diagnoses in which the other psychiatric diagnosis would also warrant hospitalization or would have a high probability of adversely complicating treatment
7   Suicidal risk, especially with a history of previous attempts
8   BAL in risky range – above 300 with minimal signs of intoxication
9   Low ego strength
10 Polydrug abuse
11 Little or no commitment to abstinence as a goal
12 Court ordered or demanded by employer as a condition for continued employment
13 Cases where denial is much stronger and more dominant than the desire for help

Advantages of hospitalization are many. Physical and psychiatric problems can be more accurately assessed and dealth with. There is enforced abstinence. Minimal brain damage, which is more the rule that the exception, has some time to begin to clear. The program is highly concentrated so that attention to recovery is a 24-hour proposition. Peer support, education, and help in working through denial and painful affects is more effective since peers get to know the patient better. Encouragement for family involvement is greater. Counselors and other professionals can concentrate their efforts. Opportunities for exercise, structured leisure time and reading are present. More attention is paid to relapse prevention. Close attention and more flexibility can be given to detoxification.

The traditional 28-day stay, developed by the craft level professionals, is not absolute. Some can successfully use a shorter stay. Generally speaking, the first week is spent just being exposed, the second week becoming interested, the third week involved and the fourth week attached. There is currently an unfortunate trend toward shorter inpatient stays, driven not by scientific evidence or clinical judgment but by economics.

14 Withdrawal and Detoxification

Since alcohol is a depressant there is a rebound excitation on cessation of chronic use, sometimes called biphasic inhibition excitation. The withdrawal syndrome can vary in degree depending on the amount and duration of drinking, nutrition, tissue tolerance, organ toxicity, age and general physiological and psychological status. CNS complications can be withdrawal seizures, DTs and hallucinosis. Various classifications of withdrawal exist.

Many alcoholics can be successfully withdrawn on an outpatient basis if there is a responsible other person to assist. Careful physical assessment should be done to rule out such things as liver disease, subdural hematoma, hidden infection, fractures, internal bleeding, etc. BALs have no place in determining hospitalization, a decision which should be based on clinical judgement of various factors.

The severity of the withdrawal syndrome varies from mild to severe. Milder withdrawal symptoms are nausea, insomnia, anxiety and general dysphoria, mild tremor, mild tachycardia, mild hypertension, anorexia and headache. Severe states include such additional things as marked tremor, sweating, hyperactivity, decreased sensory perception, confusion, moderate hypertension, moderate tachycardia and more severe dysphoria. Muscle twitching almost to a subseizure level may be present and can be prodromal to DTs or withdrawal seizures. Milder states clear within 24–36 h, severe states in 3–5 days, although it may last 7–10 days. There is such a syndrome, unfortunately not in DSM-III-R but well documented in the literature, as protracted withrawal syndrome. This occurs after severe withdrawal and in addition to the above-mentioned symptoms includes such symptoms as labile pulse and blood pressure, respiratory irregularities, depressive episodes, transient psychotic episodes, irritability, fatigue, forgetfulness, distractibility and impaired concentration. This may last from a month to as long as a year. The EEG shows decreased sleep time, decreased slow wave sleep, increased REM and increased sleep latency. This seems to be a result of a mixture of depression and an organic brain syndrome mingling with withdrawal.

The incidence of DTs, which can be life threatening, varies according to different studies on different subpopulations. Tremors, confusion, hallucinations, especially visual, and agitation are present. Withdrawal seizures occur within the first 60 h after cessation and are typically grand mal in type.

Hallucinosis, both auditory and visual, tends to be an isolated phenomenon devoid of other symptoms and occurring in a clear sensorium. It can begin several days after cessation and can last for considerable lengths of time.

Catecholamines are increased during withdrawal as a rebound phenomenon. Urinary norepinephrine (NE) and adrenaline are increased and are directly proportional to the severity of withdrawal. The γ-aminobutyric acid complex is involved in withdrawal. Magnesium can be lowered due to depression of the respiratory center resulting in respiratory alkalosis which shifts magnesium. It is also lowered from decreased intake, malabsorption and excessive renal excretion. Lowered potassium occurs for the same reasons and contributes to motor weakness, depression, exhaustion and cardiac arrhythmias. Sodium retention leads to cellular hyperirritability. Nutritional deficiencies contribute to hyperarousal. Cerebral blood flow is reduced for the first 48 h. REM is increased, and there is speculation that hallucinations may be, in part, a 'breakthrough' of this effect. Insomnia is a rebound phenomenon and may last a week or more after cessation.

Inpatient detoxification should include general measures of a private room, low light level, no visitors, allowing the patient to sleep, normal fluid intake, no smoking unless attended, checking vital signs and reassurance. The use of standardized 'routine' orders is deplorable – every patient needs individually tailored care. Routine orders cannot be geared to severity or duration of withdrawal. The use of intravenous fluids is contraindicated. There is already cellular and brain overhydration and the use of intravenous fluids prolongs detoxification and increases the risk of seizures. The only exception to this is severe malnutrition with clinical evidence of dehydration. Thiamine HCl, 100 mg, intramuscularly every 24 h for 3 doses is needed. Magnesium should not be used routinely but used only in the presence of cardiac arrhythmias or laboratory evidence of deficiency. The same guideline holds for the use of potassium. The B vitamins should be used only in the presence of malnutrition or liver disease since there is no B vitamin deficiency in most cases. B_{12} and folate levels should be checked, and B_{12} and folate used if needed. Stools for occult blood should be checked for 3 days. Total body weight should be checked daily. As noted previously serum iron drops during withdrawal due to marked uptake by a depressed bone marrow. Benzodiazepines are the drugs of choice in treating withdrawal. They are safe, cross-tolerant with alcohol, less sedating, more effective and more anxiolytic. An initial high loading dose (20 mg of diazepam or 100 mg chlordiazepoxide) repeated in 1–2 h, followed by a tailored tapering over the next 2–10 days works well. Diazepam is slightly more sedating but has slightly better antiseizure properties. In the presence of liver disease, oxazepam or lorazepam is preferable since these have no enzyme induction, no intermediate metabolites and a shorter half life. Seizures are best treated with intravenous diazepam, 5–30 mg/min. Thermal regulation can be disturbed and temperatures up to 38 °C can occur but above that are apt to be from infection. Rarely there is superthermia, with poor prognosis.

Antipsychotics are contraindicated, although haloperidol has been used for hallucinations and other psychotic symptoms. Antipsychotics lower seizure threshold, are not cross tolerant, can be toxic to the liver, give extrapyramidal side effects, alter temperature regulation, slow metabolism and are not very effective. Paraldehyde, which was commonly used in the past, has no place in treatment today. It is too sedating, can be toxic to the liver and lungs, is highly addictive, has an offensive odor, has little anticonvulsant property, and does not mix with disulfiram. Barbiturates also formerly enjoyed popularity but induce microsomal enzymes, thus competing with ETOH, have less margin of safety, and are not as effective as the benzodiazepines. If tremors do not adequately subside with benzodiazepines and magnesium the use of propanolol, 10 mg every 6 h, can be helpful, but should not be used in the presence of hallucinations, asthma or congestive heart failure.

Polydrug use will prolong alcohol detoxification, especially other sedatives and narcotics. It is not the focus of this guide to discuss other drug dependencies.

Attention to organ pathology is important and needs individual attention and treatment. Phenytoin should not be used unless there has been a pre-existing seizure disorder independent of the alcoholism. It is ineffective in withdrawal seizures and takes 2–3 days before reaching effective plasma levels of 10–20 µg.

The psychological management of the patient during detoxification is even more important than the physiologic. It is here that the initial working through of denial, a commitment to sobriety and rehabilitation, and essential linkages to treatment personnel and recovering other patients can be made. Detoxification alone without the intervention and therapy of an alcohol rehabilitation treatment team is inadequate professional care.

15 Interactions of Alcohol and Other Drugs

Interactions can be additive, potentiating or antagonistic. Indirect interactions include effects on absorption, excretion, metabolism, protein binding, distribution, and cross-tolerance. Other variables are individual variations, nutrition, speed of interactions, differences in interaction of metabolites, presence of liver damage, and unexplained side effects. Pharmacokinetics vary with age, body mass, body fat, liver and renal functions, water content, sex, gastrointestinal pH, ingestion of food, type of beverage and speed of consumption.

Congeners are other alcohols, aldehydes, ketones, phenols, acids, tannins and esters that give the beverage taste and aroma. They are more depressing to the CNS than ETOH, and are both additive and potentiating. Congener content increases progressively in this order: vodka, gin, Canadian whiskey, rum, scotch, cognac, Irish whiskey, bourbon, beer and wine. Congeners are more toxic than alcohol and slow the metabolism of alcohol.

42% of alcoholic men and 36% of alcoholic women use street drugs, often in combination. Polydrug abusers are sometimes called 'garbage heads'. The entire spectrum of other drugs is involved. Detoxification in polydrug abusers is more complicated, takes longer, and is more difficult. Opioids, with the exception of codeine, are highly addictive. 20% of methadone maintenance patients develop alcohol addiction, and this subgroup has a tenfold mortality rate. If the BAL is 180–200 mg% a therapeutic intramuscular dose of 15–30 mg of morphine sulfate can be lethal for reasons not fully understood.

Alcoholics smoke twice as much as non-alcoholics. Nicotine is mildly potentiating and alcohol increases the absorption of tobacco tars. Polydrug abusers have multiple withdrawal syndromes, more organ pathology, more aberrant behavior, more resistance to entering treatment and a poorer prognosis.

Barbiturates and non-barbiturate sedatives are potentiating. Meprobamate is highly potentiating and addictive. There is no justification for its use in the treatment of alcoholism. Paraldehyde has the greatest cross-tolerance and is potentiating. It is risky to use if the BAL is higher than 150. Chloral hydrate is potentiating, inhibits alcohol dehydrogenase (resulting in a 2–4 times increase in AcH) and accumulates. Ultran and hydroxyzine, besides being very poor anxiolytics, potentiate.

Benzodiazepines are cross-tolerant, not potentiating, antagonize the depressant effects of alcohol and have the highest safety index.

Anesthetics are additive. Alcohol prolongs induction but once induced much less anesthesia is required. The total amount of anesthesia required to cause death is one third that of non-alcoholics. These effects persist for a long time in abstinent recovering chronic alcoholics suggesting permanent cross-tolerance.

Phenothiazines, reserpine and other antipsychotics reduce liver metabolism of alcohol and vice versa. They also potentiate depression and lower seizure threshold. Their use is contraindicated for the first 48 h after cessation of ETOH.

Stimulants such as caffeine, picrotoxin and strychnine are antagonistic. Amphetamines are unpredictable. Pentylenetetrazol is antagonistic but risks producing a seizure. Methylphenidate is synergistic.

Since 75 % of the trichloroacetic acids (TCAs) are metabolized by the liver, alcoholic liver disease interferes with TCA plasma levels. Amitriptyline, nortriptyline and trimipramine potentiate, imipramine has no effect, and protriptyline and desipramine antagonize, suggesting a correlation with the sedative-stimulating spectrum of the tricyclics.

Microsomal enzyme induction increases plasma levels of phenytoin, oral anticoagulants (apt to get internal bleeding) and sulfonurea antidiabetic agents since these compete with ETOH for metabolism.

Alcohol triggers biogenic amines, including tyramine, so it is prohibited for those taking monoamine oxidase inhibitors. Monoamine oxidase inhibitors also inhibit alcohol dehydrogenase.

Diuresis from alcohol will give higher levels of lithium. Tetraethylthiuram, phenylbutazone and metronidazole inhibit AcH dehydrogenase, thus giving marked rises in blood AcH. These also give a rise in plasma catecholamines. These effects can last up to 3–4 days. The sulfonurea antidiabetics, tolbutamide, carbutamide and chlorpropamide, also produce an annoying hypersensitivity with alcohol but not to a degree that would be useful for prohibition for drinking.

β-Adrenergic blockers diminish the euphoriant effect of ETOH by inhibiting the adrenergic system. More study is needed. ETOH and digitalis will increase cardiac irritability. During detoxification this effect will be intensified if magnesium levels are low.

All chemicals which are toxic will have the toxicity increased in the presence of ETOH.

If tolerance to ETOH has developed then drugs which are cross-tolerant may be used in doses which would otherwise be excessive.

16 Dynamics of Denial

Denial is the single most important issue in dealing with the alcoholic and is the most prominent feature of the disorder. It adversely affects not only the patient but all significant others, makes the person resist getting help, influences the quality and quantity of treatment, provokes negative countertransference and promotes relapse.

Denial as used in describing a dynamic in chemical dependency is broader than the usual psychiatric definition of this defensive maneuver. The more classical definition is limited to a conscious refusal to acknowledge an obvious reality. In chemical dependency it refers to a continuum of both conscious and unconscious avoidance of facing and competently dealing with all the issues involved, such as loss of control of drinking, helplessness, guilt, shame, damaged sense of self, self-destructiveness, deleterious effects on others, morbid future, and the like. It avoids both the problem and consequences.

Denial in the chemically dependent person is used internally to deal with ego and superego warnings of the problem, and externally to deal with confrontation by others. Minimization is a subset of denial. Denial varies in degree from time to time, and varies from one area of application to another. Denial generally becomes more progressive in degree and scope as the disease progresses.

Whether the drinker is a social drinker or an alcoholic the 'pleasure principle' is served. There are secondary gains and denial is used to maintain these pleasures. Intoxication, whether minimal or severe, produces relaxation, euphoria, escape from inner conflicts, disinhibition, and forgetting of painful realities and is thus ego syntonic and serving the 'pleasure principle'. In addition, the altered states of consciousness permit a self-serving blur of being taken care of, with a resultant freedom of personal responsibility, and thus a regression to the illusion of a symbiosis with the world. How often do we see the intoxicated person inappropriately confiding personal matters to someone else as if that person was a parental figure. This further serves the 'pleasure principle'. All of this is retained as a memory paradigm for future intoxicant use.

Yet the observing self generally knows the difference between sobriety and intoxication. If there is no use of denial at this juncture then the person is more apt to maintain control over social drinking, but if denial begins to be employed then the person is at risk for progression. If the person progresses to heavy social drinking a new factor is added, namely physiological tolerance. This requires larger amounts of alcohol to serve the 'pleasure principle' dynamics just outlined, and at this point psychobiological conditioning becomes an added factor. This is a real threat to the sense of ego mastery, and denial of this insidious conditioning often creeps in. The person may still be able to maintain control at this point, but is at higher risk for progression to loss of control. The dynamic of denial is not the only factor for progression to loss of control but the intensity and scope of denial, if significant, can be crucial to progression.

With both heavy social drinking and early out of control drinking, there are adverse impacts on the self and the environment. Hangovers, withdrawal symptoms, the 'need' for a drink, the subtle deterioration in cognition and judgment, the destructiveness to family and interpersonal relationships and to work performance are all ego dystonic realities. Since all of this provokes guilt, shame, loss of self-esteem, challenges of competence, and inner pain, the person seldom seeks help at this point and usually alternates between total denial and transient periods of total abstinence, which is a form of partial denial.

When loss of control is evident a new issue is introduced – helplessness. To quote Dr. Margaret Bean-Bayog at this point:

'Repeated attempts to recover control predictably fail. This gradually destroys hope. Alcoholism destroys the person's belief he is a normal, worthwhile person, for he finds himself repeatedly behaving destructively. Self-esteem deteriorates. The experience forbids the normal social wish to be able to drink socially. The alcoholic becomes guilt ridden. He is demoralized in his attempt to solve his problem with drinking, although alcoholics almost invariably make repeated constructive attempts before they give up in despair. He does not respond to his failures by saying that he needs help because of denial, shame, fear, and confusion. The failures humiliate him and/or her, and he is afraid that if he talks about what is happening to him he will be stigmatized and his despair will be confirmed. Most people experience a diagnosis of alcoholism as a tragedy. Growing helplessness engenders regression. Efforts at problem-solving are given up. The alcoholic no longer believes in the possibility of a solution and he retreats into regression, avoidance, magical thinking and denial. As this increases he realizes he cannot stop and he is terrified of stopping knowing he would be faced with emptiness and sickness from the loss of drinking. He would also be faced with his shame and guilt, which are so intense that they are hard for most non-alcoholics to comprehend. One choice is to head for "the gutter"; another is to give it up but he does not believe he can stop. The third choice is denial.' She goes on to say, 'The general formula holds: the greater the pain and the less the hope, the more rigid the denial, and the less likelihood of successful treatment. When denial is so dysfunctional, it must be regarded as almost psychotic.'

Denial is also woven into a fifth dynamic, self-destructiveness. Primary masochism and self-destructive life styles exist in some personality disorders as a pre-existing condition prior to the onset of alcoholism but can also be a by product of alcoholism itself. Considerable secondary gain is obtained in these maneuvers. Denial is a prominent feature of these people. Secondary masochism and self-destructiveness is definitely a by-product of alcoholism. It stems from the anger at self for the inability to control drinking and a punishment of self for guilt and shame. Denial of this dynamic leads to further loss of control as a form of punishment, and thus a vicious circle ensues.

Denial enters into drinking at many levels and in many ways. Each aspect of it must be dealt with in treatment with nonjudgmental, noncritical and sympathetic understanding through repeated explanations.

Insights gained through exposure to other alcoholics and the various treatment systems provide the route for internal resolution of denial. It is much more involved than just the 'first step' in AA. Guilt, fear and narcissistic needs for omnipotence, often compulsive, need to be reduced before the person is ready for meaningful dealing with denial. Attempts by others to confront denial when accusatory, manipulative or aggressive are usually counterproductive. Another type of behavior commonly found in alcoholics is what is called the 'con game'. Deliberate falsifications, denial and/or minimization of drinking and intentional distortion of other issues are often used by alcoholics to manipulate others so as to avoid unpleasantries or coverup aberrant behavior. This can become so frequent as to become habitual and a way of life that is used even when not necessary. This life style complicates the issues. An element of denial, both conscious and unconscious, provokes this conning. This is to be seen as partially compulsive to avoid rejection as well as having secondary gains. Abstinent alcoholics are often aware that they no longer 'con' people.

17 Intervention

An alcoholic seldom seeks help voluntarily. Intervention is the term given to the process of persuading the alcoholic to voluntarily seek treatment. Court orders or employer ultimatums are not considered interventions, although these can be effective. Usually someone close to the person prods the patient to seek help, often associated with a current crisis. If the patient resists prompting there is a highly effective method of ganging up on him by a group using emotional appeals which has the name 'intervention'. This is a skilled approach directed by a person trained in the technique. It consists of the interventionist gathering all the significant others, family, friends, neighbors, boss, etc., in separate preliminary sessions without the patient. These people are asked to collect hard data on dates, level of intoxication and consequences. At a subsequent meeting in the interventionist's office these same people, this time with the patient, confront the patient with the facts. This is done without anger or bitterness and in as loving a way as possible with the final appeal of asking the patient to surrender to getting help. The interventionist instructs the people ahead of time on how to present and he orchestrates the order of presentation, progressively going from the least to the most affectively important person to the patient. Ultimatums, such as divorce, loss of job, etc., are used only if all else fails, but must be sincere and must be effected if the intervention fails.

18 Employee Assistance Programs

Primarily to deal with alcoholism in industry, special people are designated to expedite treatment and rehabilitation. These are known as Employer Assistance Personnel. They have now begun to be involved in a wider range of problems than just alcoholism, but still interface with treatment systems and are even members of the treatment teams in some facilities. They do more than act as an interventionist but assist employees and families in a number of ways. They often get to know the employee rather well and can even become a significant other. They provide counseling, ombudsmanship, give support, act as role models, assist with reintegration in the work place, work out reassignments, and are excellent history takers. They will often visit hospitalized patients and are helpful in discharge planning. They also are constructive in impacting favorable and more humane corporate policies toward alcoholism. Some are full time, some are available to industry and business on a part-time basis. Many have had professional training and experience in counseling.

19 Dual Diagnoses

This terminology is given when alcoholism exists with other DSM-III-R psychiatric diagnoses. Incidence data varies from study to study but are probably at least 60%. Some studies have indicated much higher figures. The author's survey of 550 admissions with the primary diagnosis of alcoholism to a private psychiatric hospital with 45 staff psychiatrists revealed additional psychiatric diagnoses on the face sheet in 51%. Admittedly, this survey was not quality controlled.

Polydrug abuse is common, especially in adolescents and young adults, 42% of young adult males and 36% of females were polydrug abusers in one study. Some have other drugs as their drug of choice, some use other drugs occasionally but use alcohol as their first choice, some use alcohol when their other drug is not available, and some use alcohol to potentiate or ameliorate the effects of other drugs. Drug intoxication, especially from amphetamines, lysergic acid and phencyclidine, can mimic schizophrenia. Blood and urine drug screens are quite useful, although a positive result for marijuana can sometimes occur in chronic heavy users 7 days after cessation since it is stored in fat. The sensitivity of the laboratory test for marijuana needs to be considered. Polydrug abuse usually involves lengthier and more complex detoxification, with the exception of marijuana, and requires more attention in rehabilitation. Narcotics Anonymous and Cocaine Anonymous, modeled after AA, are appropriate.

Axis I Disorders

Further studies are needed to look at the prevalence of these disorders in subpopulations of alcoholics. There is probably no greater prevalence of alcoholism in middle and upper class schizophrenics, but there does seem to be more in the indigent schizophrenics. Affective disorders seem to have a higher prevalence, especially in women, who have a higher prevalence rate of secondary alcoholism. Also alcoholic women have higher rates of depression. When affective disorders are present a careful history is needed to determine, when possible, whether the disorder anteceded the alcoholism. It is, incidentally, diagnostically erroneous to diagnose depression and alcoholism on admission to treatment when the person has been drinking. Almost all drinking alcoholics are clinically depressed as a by product of alcohol. This clears within a few days to a week or two, and does not require antidepressant medication. If it persists beyond this period of time then consider either an atypical depression or other forms of depression. These do warrant antidepressant medication.

Cocaine users often get depressed during detoxification and sometimes for months afterwards and often will have chronic or recurring depression for up to a year or more of abstinence. This should definitely by treated with antidepressant medication. Antidepressant medication has also been found to be statistically useful in relapse prevention for cocaine. Prescriptions for antidepressants should be time limited. Clinical judgment as to whether to use them at all should be heavily weighed by factors such as therapeutic alliance, progress in rehabilitation and linkage with support systems.

Psychotics should not generally be put in rehabilitation programs but should be treated individually as they would be treated otherwise. Those psychotics unable to abstain from alcohol should be placed in long-term protected environments. The current 'revolving door' of brief repeated hospitalizations for alcoholic psychotic indigents is an unacceptable quality of care and is deplorable.

The persistence of anxiety after detoxification is frequent. A careful diagnostic assessment is needed to differentiate between manipulativeness, a transient anxiety disorder provoked by the breakthrough of repressed conflicts and the loss of euphoria, a protracted withdrawal syndrome or unrelated co-existing Axis I anxiety disorder. Benzodiazepines are strongly contraindicated for these. One does not substitute one addiction for another. Buspirone, antidepressants, relaxation techniques and psychotherapy are appropriate.

Lithium is appropriate in treatment and prophylaxis of those with recurrent unipolar or bipolar depression. Again, family education and therapy are indicated in the presence of dual diagnoses. It is important in psychotherapy to look at the interactions of alcohol and other psychopathology.

Attention deficit disorder, residual type, is not rare in alcoholics, and in stimulant and cocaine abusers.

Axis II Disorders

Axis II disorders are very common. Schuckit noted that perhaps as high as 37% of alcoholic males and 27% of females have antisocial personalities. These have an 80% rate of family history positive for alcoholism, are alcoholic at an earlier age, have a more severe degree of disease, are disruptive to programs, and have an extremely poor prognosis. Borderlines and dependents are also more vulnerable. Therapy of Axis II disorders generally is that as used for non-alcoholics. As generally observed, schizoids and obsessives are not good group psychotherapy candidates.

Those with physical disease who also abuse alcohol have probably no higher prevalence than non-abusers with the exception of those with chronic pain. Chronic pain patients who abuse alcohol should be advised that alcohol is ineffective, has risky side effects, may worsen neuritis, and only adds a second problem. Those whose physical disease is aggravated by alcohol abuse, e.g., hypertensives, cardiacs, diabetics, hypothyroids, etc., should be cautioned not to use it at all. Those with chronic insomnia and iatrogenic sedative abuse may use alcohol to excess either in combination or as a substitute. These people usually have co-existing psychiatric problems and need diagnosis and treatment.

20 Treatment Models of Rehabilitation

Unfortunately, approximately 80–85% of alcoholics get no treatment. There are three models of professional rehabilitation programs.

The *Craft* model, which grew out of AA, uses alcoholism counselors, many of whom are recovering alcoholics themselves, to conduct individual and group education and counseling. They developed the traditional 28-day inpatient care, primarily empirically. There are many such centers throughout the US. Their goals are abstinence and linkage with AA. In recent years alcoholism counselors have developed credentialling standards. Counselors are usually most skillful in helping with alcoholism but are untrained in dual diagnoses and in unconscious psychic processes. Medical consultants are called in for physical problems.

The *Medical* model uses the Craft model as a base, but adds to it by having a physician as the team leader. The doctor manages detoxification, any organ pathology, and provides counseling.

The *Psychiatric* model, which is the cutting edge of the field, uses the Craft and Medical models as a base but adds psychiatric diagnosis and treatment. Individual, couples, group and family therapy will be used by the psychiatrist, singly or in combination, to diagnose and treat dual diagnoses and personality dynamics as well as provide counseling for problems in living and maintenance of sobriety. The psychiatrist also conducts continuing education for the whole treatment team in psychodynamics and in dual diagnoses.

If treatment is outpatient it should be conducted at least once a week, preferably more, for several months and preferably a year. Both individual and group therapies are used for patients and families. Inpatient treatment should be 3–4 weeks, geared to the patient's progress, and followed up with 2½–12 months of 'aftercare' by counselors and physicians on a weekly basis. Outpatient visits to the physician should be individually tailored to the treatment plan. There are two common problems seen in inpatient care: (1) denial, which takes time to work through, and which is best addressed by fellow patients and counselors, has to be dealt with gently, patiently and kindly, and (2) cognitive impairment, often more severe than it appears on the surface, which may persist for several weeks or longer. The physician should know how to test for this. It usually clears in time. Patients often grasp the presented material but do not retain it, so repetition of themes is needed.

AA should be an integral component in rehabilitation programs. Many are built around it. AA meetings, both in and out of the facility, are often mandatory in programs, although a few patients resist. Linkages with AA sponsors is important in inpatient discharge planning.

21 Rehabilitation: A Psychiatric Model

Once detoxification has been completed and the patient is mentally clear, then the long process of rehabilitation can be initiated.

The very first step, often not given sufficient attention, is the development of a therapeutic alliance and the formulation of a treatment contract. This contract should be clearly stated and should contain at least three basic points: (1) abstinence; (2) agreement to attend AA or other self-help support groups, and (3) agreement to call the therapist or sponsor at times of temptation to relapse instead of using the chemical. Some centers use written contracts.

The goals of rehabilitation are abstinence, replacing unhealthy with healthy peer groups, learning to identify and more appropriately handle affects, resolve denial, guilt and fear, relapse prevention plans, family reorganization, and growth in interpersonal skills. There can be an identity change from the negative of being an alcoholic to the positive of a recovering.

Elements of the Treatment Plan

Whether the patient is a formal or informal partner in the treatment plan depends on the clinical judgment of the therapist. Motivation for participation and levels of sophistication and psychological mindedness are important variables. The basic elements are the following.

1 Continued focus by the treatment team and peer group on inner motivation for change. Most patients have been coerced into treatment, have little desire for change, and maintain a secret desire to return to drinking, often clinging to the delusion they can control it. Self-motivation must replace external pressures for changes if treatment is to succeed.

2 Education on the scientific details of substance abuse, the effects on the mind and body, family, career, etc., is one of the core elements in rehabilitation. Education on steps to recovery are important not only to give hope but to convey the message of the disease model and healthy role models.

3 Increasing knowledge of the various secondary gains of substance abuse, e.g., relief of tension, escape from conflict, transient euphoria, release of inhibitions, means of expressing hostility, both toward self and others, excuse for aberrant behavior, entitlement to pleasure, substitute gratification, maintenance of sense of omnipotence, etc., add to the educational component.

4 Education on how to handle problems of living without resorting to chemicals is essential to relapse prevention. This focuses on both intrapersonal and interpersonal functioning.

5 How to use support systems and how to develop attachments and positive feedback loops with these is integral to AA, to counter omnipotence, narcissism and denial, and to growth. Such support systems include self-help groups, sponsors, family, therapists, employee assistance personnel.

6 Formulation of an emergency plan for unanticipated stress and temptations is also a part of relapse prevention.

7 Family involvement in education about the disease, resolution of conflicts, relearning of healthy family systems, and support of the patient is a must whenever possible.

8 Long-term follow-up and help with positive reinforcement, role modeling and personality growth is as important as abstinence.

A structured rehabilitation program initially inolves a planned day of education, support, peer involvement, self-help support groups, such as AA and NA, family participation and individual counseling. This is best done in a therapeutic community where all the patients are chemically dependent and the community is led by trained alcoholism and substance abuse counselors.

Such a community affords both peer and professional pressure to look at denial, faulty patterns of affective and inter-personal management, motivation for change and targeted goals for change. There should be a focus not just on the goal of abstinence but also on learning healthy and mature patterns of living. Individual psychotherapy by the attending psychiatrist may well be needed when resistances to a natural progression of improvement is significant or when areas of significant psychiatric psychopathology impede progress. The attending psychiatrist otherwise focuses on education and physical problems.

The importance of family involvement in rehabilitation cannot be over-emphasized. Families are always involved and it is well known that chemical dependency is a family disease. No typical patterns of pathology have been found, so each family must be studied as to the pathology involved. A systems approach here is most useful as well as a psychodynamic under-standing of conflict and interpersonal patterns. Education and involvement of families should be individual, in groups, and whenever possible also at times with the identified patient. Whenever subspecialists in family counseling can be found these should be utilized. While education on chemical dependency lends itself to groups of families, it is best to deal with specific family psychopathology on an individual family basis. The family subspecialist should be aware of when to request help from the attending psychiatrist to deal with more deep-seated issues.

Rehabilitation has been divided into early, middle and late phases since the issues and management are somewhat different in each.

Early Phase

As patients are first being exposed to education and new learning about self and others, there is a steady exposure to the concepts of the disease model. This lends hope and somewhat defuses guilt and shame over loss of control. Peer exposure not only counters the sense of aloneness and uniqueness but also lends powerful opportunities for new attachments, role modeling and support. Simple confrontations of the problems and the promise of change without moral judgments is the best ambience. One caveat is not to seriously challenge defenses, such as denial, rationalization, minimization, etc., too vigorously. Healthier modes of functioning need to be found first before much can be done with insights that raise anxiety. Patients are in a great deal of pain already, although they may not disclose it because of being too embarrassed. Zimberg has said that the patient in this stage senses the idea 'I can't drink'.

It is important to understand that the patient at the end of this first stage is still very fragile and vulnerable to relapse and therefore needs a great deal of external support and control. Planned aftercare meetings as an outpatient with the counselor on a weekly basis, AA meetings 4–6 times a week, and weekly outpatient contacts with the attending psychiatrist for a 10- to 12-week period is recommended as a minimum. The focus of these sessions is still supportive, positive reinforcement and identification of healthy modes of functioning.

The end objective of this first phase is the establishment of some inner controls which all concerned have a concensus on.

Middle Phase

When internal controls have been reasonably established and the patient volunteers confidence in these, then the middle phase begins. At this point problems and conflicts that have been put aside earlier because of being too emotionally charged and also because of being secondary to the primary issue of abstinence are often brought up, usually by the patient whenever there has been a good therapeutic alliance. In fact, the spontaneous volunteering of these matters by the patient is a good indication of a good therapeutic alliance and positive transference. These issues can be general or specific or can be oriented toward healing or toward growth, or both. New ways of handling feelings, appropriate assertiveness, coping with anger, handling failures and frustrations, structuring leisure time, being comfortable with support groups and partnerships, learning to handle stress and relax more are common general issues. Specific inner problems such as distortions in self-image, chronic hostilities, fears of trusting and of emotional intimacy, learned helplessness, sexual conflicts and other inner conflicts are quite common. These invariably are stress producing to the individual and to others around the individual.

Individual, conjoint, group, family, and sex therapy are treatment modalities best tailored by the clinical judgment of the attending psychiatrist.

Behavioral approaches such as stress management, assertiveness training, social skills building and the like are useful, but should be utilized on a prescription basis according to needs and appropriateness.

In general, it is still not advisable to interpret transference or to uncover unconscious conflicts in psychotherapy during this phase. The ego still needs considerable support and the person is still too vulnerable to relapse. Should relapses occur the therapist should be alert to negative countertransference and should view the relapse as a signal to re-evaluate the dynamic issues involved.

This middle phase usually takes 6 months to a year. Blane considers these goals as the end of the middle phase: (1) spontaneous engagement in new activities, interests and behavior; (2) handles unique, potentially conflictual situations in an adult and self-satisfying manner; (3) accepts set backs without becoming anxious or depressed, or without acting out; (4) knows and experiences feelings as they occur, and (5) when conflicted, examines and works through the conflict himself or in a nondefensive way with the therapist.

Late Phase
Patients can either terminate therapy at the end of the middle phase or can go on to uncovering, psychoanalytically or

cognitively oriented psychotherapy. Patients with definite personality or sexual conflicts are potential candidates for uncovering psychotherapy. Stable sobriety, however, must have been well established.

It is also axiomatic that the chemically dependent person must have abstinence as a life-long standard. Life-long utilization of self-help groups is not only valuable for maintaining abstinence but offers opportunities for personality use, addressed in the section on the Psychodynamics of AA.

Role Models

If the therapist is not a recovering person then it is important for the patient to have a mature recovering other person to relate to on an on-going basis. This role model can be a sponser or other 'recovering' who befriends the patient. It is important for the non-recovering therapist to encourage and support this role modeling. It becomes something not only useful to the patient as an ego ideal but it affords the patient the opportunity to have a realization of self-worth by becoming a role model for others.

22 Psychotherapy

General Remarks

During the first phase one should generally avoid discussing dynamics that were etiologic. Alcoholics, especially in the initial stages of recovery, are often curious about the reasons for their drinking. Therapists should avoid this until much later since they are very apt to use these as reasons to 'explain' the problem and avoid self-examination rather than examine the whole picture. Once sobriety has been reasonably well established these can be gone into if the patient still wishes to know.

The psychotherapist should give equal priority to the maintenance of sobriety as to emphasis on other issues, such as dual diagnoses. Even if later on there is more intensive psychotherapy of inner conflicts, the alcoholism should not be lost sight of.

Those who are not motivated, are unable to establish a therapeutic alliance, have antisocial personality or organic brain damage are not good psychotherapy candidates.

Psychotherapy enhances recovery rates of rehabilitation programs and vice versa. Areas of focus are given in the following.

Attention to Sobriety

This should be directive inquiries into experiences and participation in AA, avoidance of drinking buddies, relapse prevention, use of sponsor, progress in resolution of denial, impulse control, attitudes toward drinking, importance of continued treatment, improvement in getting in touch with affects, changes in family and job functioning, new pleasures, exercise, energy, other substance abuse, changes in self-image, moods, dealing with the loss of drinking pleasures, craving, use of leisure time, etc. Slips are to be expected and should be dealt with as a learning experience.

Psychodynamic

1   Supportive, individual, conjoint, group and family therapy are used. More will be discussed later about family issues. The same psychotherapy of a supportive and counseling nature given with non-alcoholics is used here concerning problems in living, behavior, interpersonal issues, anxiety, dysphoria, importance of honesty, etc.

Group therapy is usually better than individual for the overly dependent, avoidant, narcissistic, histrionic, milder obsessive compulsive more stable borderline personalities and those with pre-existing low self-esteem. Schizoid and paranoid personalities as well as unstable borderlines and obsessive compulsives do better individually.

2   Conflict oriented. There is an abundance of psychopathology both in dual diagnosis and with characterologic abnormalities seen in alcoholics. In fact some studies have concluded that this exists in 100% of cases. Orthodox psychoanalysis is contraindicated because of its anxiety-provoking tendency but psychoanalytically oriented psychotherapy and all other dynamic psychotherapies are useful. It should be utilized if the patient is seriously interested and motivated and/or the conflicts clearly impair the recovery process. Adequate ego strength and psychological mindedness affect selection criteria. Positive transferences seldom require interpretation since patients may return for further therapy at some future time but negative and erotic transferences do need active intervention. The resolution of conflicts is not to be considered as treatment of the walking well, but an important and often essential element in the treatment of the full spectrum of this disease.

Most alcoholics respond to psychotherapy, and treatment of many is rewarding and enjoyable for the therapist.

23 Alcoholics Anonymous

A Behavioral Science View of the AA System

AA is an integral element in treatment. It was the first approach that had proven success. It began in the 1930s, has a large membership and has world-wide activity. For some it may be the only treatment needed. Its 12 steps and 12 principles are well established.

While it is appropriate to see each person as unique and to formulate the pathology of the problem drinker in individualized variations of emphasis, there has nonetheless been a clinical consensus of the commonality of certain affective issues and psychodynamics of the problem drinker. Many may be conceptualized as secondary to uncontrolled drinking, by-products if you will, but then becoming significantly influential in overall interpersonal behavior and in contributing to further loss of control. Once the spiral has begun, it is difficult to stop. Some of these dynamics may of course be antecedent to the loss of control but once the discontrol has ensued there is a vicious circle of disturbed world (both inner and outer) – alcoholism – disturbed world – alcoholism.

The following dynamic issues are common to most alcoholics: denial; self-destructiveness; pathological narcissism (all alcoholics put self first); loss of self-respect; guilt and shame; the insult that loss of control gives to the sense of ego mastery ('I'm not too drunk to drive'); the desire to return to controlled drinking with all of its ego syntonic pleasures and the illusion of symbiosis; alienation from others; demoralization; suppression and repression of painful affects and memories; helplessness, and hopelessness. The defense mechanisms of denial, rationalization, minimization and projection are common.

Where does AA come in? It cuts through the defenses and points immediately to two crucial points: (a) challenge to narcissism, denial, rationalization ('You can't fool us – we've been there'), and (b) alienation, guilt and shame ('We don't condemn, we know how to help, we want to help, and we have proven answers').

How Does AA Work?

As helplessness and powerlessness over alcohol, the first step, is seen as a reality then there can be receptiveness to the idea that external factors can be helpful in recovery.

Control of drinking is seen for the first time by the subject as neither totally the individual's responsibility nor the responsibility of others but a shared responsibility because of accepting that a 'higher power', i.e., influences outside oneself, is needed. This sharing is via interdependence. This sort of adult interdependence is not only a healthy model for the problem of alcohol control but for human relatedness in general. So AA becomes not only a method to achieve sobriety but a source of new attachments and remodeling. Working through the 12 steps gives perspective to the problems and a sense of accomplishment. Through listening to others there can be less isolation, more understanding of denial and guilt, a sense of 'undoing' past transgressions, and a sense of commonality and belongingness. Peer support provides acceptance, equalization, role modeling, non-judgmental confession and further reminders of the gravity of the disease. The lack of rules and hierarchy encourages spontaneity and humility. Tokens and 'birthdays' give recognition, a sense of accomplishment and pride. Sobriety takes on a positive identity. Sponsors are helpful for relapse prevention. The opportunity to help others helps resolve guilt and promotes self-esteem. Group experiences may help those who are timid or lacking in social skills. The 12 traditions provide a sense of organization, substance, belongingness and pride.

Caveats

It is most important for the alcoholic to find a group where there is a 'fit'. A professional person, for example, will feel out of place in a blue collar group. Some are uncomfortable with the religious emphasis and others become bored with repetitious 'drunkalogues'. Some misconceptions are still widespread in many groups, such as the admonition not to take any 'mind-altering drugs' including antipsychotics, antidepressants, lithium, etc., or the myth that concurrent dual psychiatric diagnoses are always by-products of drinking. Some AA groups, unfortunately, are hostile toward psychiatry. The frequent dense clouds of tobacco smoke at meetings is also objectionable.

AA is not for everyone and the person should not be chided for not going if they have valid objections. The drop out rate is high and the success rate only modest, but, nonetheless, it works for many and should be offered to all.

Allied Groups

AlAnon, Alateen, Alatot, Narcotics Anonymous, Cocaine Anonymous, etc., are well established and useful, both for the alcoholic as well as the family.

24 Family

Alcoholism is often defined as a family disease since it puts a major stress on families with profound effects. In fact, sometimes family members are termed 'co-alcoholic'. Claudia Beck said, 'Alcoholism is dominoes. The alcohol knocks down the alcoholic who knocks down everyone including themselves.'

Families can be seen at four levels of functioning: functional, neurotically enmeshed, chaotic and broken. Triangulating families wherein each uses another to communicate with the primary object have a higher rate of alcoholism. Female alcoholics tend to marry male alcoholics but not vice versa. Opposites, e.g., hysterics and obsessives, tend to marry each other. The notion that a woman marries an alcoholic for neurotically predetermined motives is an outmoded myth. There are no personality differences between the wives of alcoholics and non-alcoholics. Some alcoholics are closet drinkers and able to hide their drinking but not the effects.

Alcoholism is devastating to families. Damage is done by intoxicated behavior, the effects of alcoholism on personality functioning and by pre-existing pathological personality functioning. All are interwoven. The alcoholic is not infrequently abusive, sexually and physically, given to destructive rages, sexually unfaithful, sexually obnoxious, sexually impotent, reckless and irresponsible with money, involved with the police, embarrassing and in general difficult to live with. Wives withdraw or attack, or both, and children withdraw. Alcoholism is both cause and effect of disturbances in family functioning. There are no basic differences between non-alcoholics and alcoholics in conflicted marriages other than compounding of problems in the alcoholic. Husbands of female alcoholics are less accepting and less willing to consider it a disease and more apt to leave. The alcoholic's irresponsibility, impulsiveness, unpredictability, acting out, self-centeredness, inadequacies, recklessness and rebelliousness adversely influence family life. Sometimes the alcoholic tries to recruit his wife into drinking and if she agrees, in an attempt to control his drinking, then the problem progresses.

Alcoholism becomes interactional with neuroticisms which then become involved in feedback loops between all family members, provoking more anxiety, frustration, anger, hopelessness and power struggles. Denial and punishment are resorted to. Defense mechanisms of all kinds are mobilized. Who is in control becomes intensified and often ends in stalemate. Wives are often driven to having to assume more responsibility and are then falsely accused of being dominant. If the family does not progressively deteriorate to the point of chaos and disintegration then a certain leveling off of family functioning at an operational, but highly neurotic, level to preserve homeostasis will occur, but the alcoholic continues his drinking. The dynamics in this homeostasis permit the alcoholic to continue the drinking, and in fact may even require the drinking to maintain the homeostasis. The Craft level professionals call such members 'enablers'. At this point there is resistance to change by all and there is a hidden bargain to maintain the system. The effects of this are not only felt by the alcoholic and the family but by the extended family and society. Anger and bitterness become dominating themes, and no one wins.

Family education on alcoholism is an integral part of rehabilitation, and family psychotherapy, individual or in family groups of 5–7, has been found to be the best approach yet. It should always be combined with individual therapy and AA systems. It is not to be used with chaotic or broken families and should not be used with psychotics, multiple drug users or antisocial personalities. It focuses on studying feedback dynamics amongst all family members. It is important not to scapegoat or overly focus on any one member. There are no comprehensive treatment techniques but it is best done by those professionals experienced in family therapy. Boundaries between generations, which have been blurred by alcohol, need clarification. Blaming should be avoided. The focus is on insights, education, consciousness raising and support. Termination should be open ended. The goals are education, repair of damage, forgiveness, resolution of hostility and fear, instillation of hope, rewarding positive changes, resolution of pathological homeostasis, and personal growth. Family therapy is essential with adolescents. Its use with the elderly is primarily in those whose alcoholism antedated the age of 65.

25 Disulfiram (Antabuse)

In 1937 Williams noted that rubber factory workers were hypersensitive to alcohol and traced this to exposure to tetramethylthiuram disulfide. In 1948 Hald and Jacobsen identified a congener, tetraethylthiuram disulfiram, as the factor, and this has been manufactured with the name disulfiram (Antabuse) and used as a prophylaxis for drinking.

It has no action by itself and is inert except when mixed with alcohol when there is a hypersensitivity reaction which is most unpleasant. Mild reactions occur with as low a BAL as 10 mg%/100 ml, moderate reactions with a BAL of 50–100 and severe reactions with a BAL over 125.

What is known about its metabolism does not fully account for all the reactions. It inhibits both alcohol and AcH dehydrogenases with a resultant enormous rise in circulating AcH lasting for several hours. These are zinc-containing enzymes and disulfiram chelates zinc. In the presence of liver disease there is more zinc depletion so the disulfiram reaction is heightened. There is also a marked NE release with resultant stimulation of NE systems, partly from the effects of AcH and partly a direct effect. Acetylcholine is increased giving further NE release. Tolerance does not develop and in fact is diminished (reverse tolerance) with time. It blocks dopamine-β-oxidase with a resultant increase in dopamine. It comes out in the breath as carbon disulfide.

Mild reactions are those of nausea, vomiting, flushing, headache and dysphoria. Moderate reactions additionally include sweating, thirst, chest pains, dyspnea, tachycardia, hypotension, weakness, syncope, vertigo, injected sclerae, blurred vision, hyperventilation and drowsiness. Severe reactions can additionally cause confusion, cardiovascular collapse, myocardial infarctions, seizures and death. Toxic reactions can include cardiac arrhythmias, optic neuritis, peripheral neuropathy, urticaria, gastrointestinal disturbances, hepatotoxicity and delirium. Mild and moderate reactions last 1–2 h. The drug takes 3–4 days to clear after cessation.

Medical screening should be done prior to prescribing, especially to rule out cardiac, liver or kidney pathology. Patients should carry a card with them that is an alert to their taking the drug. Patients do better if they fully understand the drug and sign a written contract.

The dosage of disulfiram should be 250 or 125 mg/day. A test dose of alcohol is not necessary. It takes 4 days for the drug to reach adequate blood levels because of slow metabolism. Treatment of severe reactions and toxic reactions is with intravenous antihistamines, intravenous vitamin C and ephedrine, plus general supportive measures. Reactions from alcohol can be up to 4 days after drug cessation. Patients should be cautioned to avoid alcoholic vinegars, cough syrups with an alcohol base, shaving lotions containing alcohol.

Disulfiram is contraindicated in the presence of coronary artery disease. Isoniazid will give toxic effects. Caution should be used with diabetes mellitus, organic brain syndrome, hypothyroidism, and epilepsy. High levels of phenytoin will occur. Metronidazole (Flagyl) gives similar effects as disulfiram, and can be substituted for disulfiram (although not as effective) but should not be used simultaneously.

Disulfiram is not used very frequently and should not be a substitute for rehabilitation and psychotherapy. It does have a place when other approaches have failed in those with a history of repeated relapses respite treatment, and in the first 6 months of outpatient treatment when this is the initial approach and prognosis is guarded. Disulfiram is often discouraged by AA. It is still a crutch and sometimes impairs full involvement in rehabilitation. Compliance rates are dismal.

26 Other Treatment Modalities

Operant conditioning, primarily the contributions of psychologists, may be useful. This includes techniques such as countering cues to drink, self-monitoring logs, cognitive rituals for dealing with risks, reinforcing systems for awareness of consequently, etc.

Behavioral modification approaches such as relaxation techniques, social skills training, assertiveness training, marital skills training and written contracts have their place.

Social services and vocational rehabilitation are useful when appropriate and when accepted by the patient.

Aversion treatment, which enjoyed modest popularity many years ago as a primary treatment approach, is still used today by very few centers. The general experience has been that results are short lived. It consists of repeatedly giving an aversive stimulus with a measured dose of alcohol until Pavlovian conditioning occurs. Aversive stimuli can be emetics (e.g., ipecac, emetine), electric shocks, succinylcholine (giving transient respiratory paralysis). These are not without some physical risks.

27 Children of Alcoholics

10 % of children under the age of 20 are in alcoholic families. It is always traumatic for children and no child escapes unscathed. These children are victimized and have long-term personality problems. It is not unusual to obtain histories not only of dysfunctional families but of child abuse and incest. While each child is unique in the amount of damage received, there are two generalizations which are ubiquitous: the problems persist, and the psychopathology becomes rigid and fixed.

To give a sense of flavor concerning these the brief description by Dr. Ruth Fox in 1956 is partially quoted: ' ... the sense of security so necessary to the building of a strong and independent ego is rarely found in the household. The child can be utterly bewildered by the sudden shift in behavior of the alcoholic. A parent who is often affectionate, understanding and funloving when sober may become morose, demanding, unreasonable, touchy, noisy and even cruel and violent when drunk. Or a naturally reserved and somewhat withdrawn parent may become sloppily sentimental and seductive in the early stages of a drinking bout, or hilariously and embarassingly exuberant. He or she may spend money wildly and make extravagant promises which are impossible to fulfill. The frequent swing from high hopes to shattering disappointments may build up in the child such a basic distrust that all his later intimate relationships will be distorted.'

Developmental pathology often seen in children are problems in forming primary relationships, delayed physical and emotional development, various expressions of anxiety, anxiousness to please others, withdrawal, lack of creativity, social

---

isolation, poor impulse control, pseudomaturation, shyness, mistrust, confusion, guilt by association, hopelessness, insecurity, excessive anger, etc. They often feel they are to blame and will adopt stereotyped roles to counteract this. Even cognitive and physical development can be retarded. They are often only spectators in their worlds rather than full participants. Pathological role models for identification promote poor communication, suppression and repression of painful affects, self-centeredness, the notion that all interpersonal relationships are power struggles, self-indulgence and narcissistic management of impulse control. A common construct is that communication is effected behaviorally not verbally, leading to acting out. There is a higher incidence of alcohol problems, childhood anxiety disorders, conduct disorders and conflicts with authority. Repressed and suppressed feelings are hurt, shame, guilt, anger, embarrassment, fear, uncertainty, mistrust, frustration, hopelessness, insecurity anxiety, loneliness, pain, and despair.

The oldest child often attempts to be an adult too soon and become hyperresponsible.

These scars not infrequently persist into adulthood and we see a constellation of personality maladaptation. Common among these effects are compulsive approval seeking, guilt feelings, low self-esteem, perfectionistic pursuits in order to gain a sense of mastery, fear of criticism, suppression and repression of feelings, shallowness in relating to people, marital isolation, overdependency, preoccupation with self, dysfunctional attitudes toward alcohol, attraction to weakness in others, fear of authority, sense of inadequacy, masochistic and sadistic themes, and lack of basic trust in intimate interpersonal relationships. In many respects they have a need-fear dilemma – they need so much of what they have never had but are afraid to ask.

There is a growing national support group, Adult Children of Alcoholics. This is an outstanding group and can often be used as an 'admission ticket' to getting professional help as well as a continuing support group for growth, destigmatization, anxiety reduction and education.

28 Alcohol and the Fetus

Damage to the fetus from maternal drinking has been known for millenia. Carthage and Sparta had laws prohibiting newly married couples from drinking. Aristotle wrote about it. Laws were passed in England 250 years ago during the gin epidemic. It can be seen in experimental animals.

Between 5 and 10% of pregnant women drink to excess. Different studies have shown incidences between 2.5 and 40%. There are possibly relationships between the amounts of consumption and the trimesters used. The full blown fetal alcohol syndrome identified in 1981 by the Fetal Alcohol Study Group of the Research Society on Alcoholism developed strict criteria for diagnosis: (1) pre- or postnatal growth retardation below the tenth percentile for gestational age; (2) CNS involvement with symptoms of neurological abnormality, developmental delay, or intellectual impairment, and (3) characteristic facial dysmorphology with at least 2 of the 3 signs, microcephaly, microphthalmia and/or shortened palpebral fissures, poorly developed philtrum, thin upper lip or flattening of the maxillary area of the upper lip. Abnormalities which do not meet the above criteria are known as fetal alcohol effects and may include deafness, teratology of the extremities, cardiac defects, oral defects, kidney and urinary tract abnormalities, liver abnormalities, immune deficiencies, hemangiomas, hirsutism and various tumors. Alterations in motor performance, reflexes, autonomic regulation and normal development also occur. All of these may be threshold related. There has even been the withdrawal syndrome in newborns in mothers who have continued to drink up until labor. The very heavy drinkers have 32% of their infants with congenital malformations. Almost all organs can be affected. Those organs with the most rapid growth are more vulnerable. Malnourishment is common. There is also a higher percentage of spontaneous abortions.

Metabolic acidosis, EEG slowing and decreased amplitude, and a sheet of aberrant neural and glial tissue covering part of the brain can be found.

The threshold between the level of alcohol use and fetal damage has not been established. The only safe guideline is total abstinence during pregnancy.

29 Outcome

It used to be thought and taught that alcoholism had an inexorably progressive downhill course that, unless interrupted, ended in death. While there are still some where that is the case, most have varying courses. Some have lengthy periods of abstinence and many have varying degrees of abuse over time. Some drink daily, some in sprees, some both. George Vaillant has done a super study to clearly demonstrate the wide variability of the course of the disease. The only ones where reasonable certainty of prognosis can be made are the skid row alcoholics. Some alcoholics stop without outside help, some stop with AA alone, and some stop only with formal rehabilitation programs. Prognosis is improved with progressively more extensive and sophisticated treatment. Varying statistics are quoted regarding success rates. Those often quoted by AA are overestimated but useful in promoting attendance. Many studies are scientifically invalid because of not being scientifically rigorous and/or being less than 24 months duration. In addition, studies have looked only at half the problem, abstinence, and not at personal functioning. Nonetheless, alcoholism is a treatable disease.

Relapses are common, almost to be expected. If the person is in continued treatment these are usually brief. Relapses should be viewed as diagnostic challenges to uncover dynamics, which should then be dealt with in treatment. Lengthy relapses often betray a lack of full commitment to treatment, sociopathy, or a feigning of involvement in rehabilitation. Many health insurance policies will cover only 2 or 3 rehabilitation programs in a lifetime, some only one.

Alcoholics should not be held fully accountable for abstinence. Remember, it is a disease. Negative and critical attitudes on the part of others are counter productive by intensifying guilt, same, fear, anger, helplessness and hopelessness. It is not uncommon to find physicians who still today are unkind to, scornful of and punitive toward alcoholics, thus adding iatrogenic factors to relapse. A more subtle factor negatively impinging on treatment is the unconscious negative counter-transference of professionals from a fundamentalist religious background.

Suicide is always a risk in alcoholics. The lifetime prevalence of suicide in the general population is 1 % but approximately 15–20 % in alcoholics. Alcohol is associated with 50 % of all suicides, whether the person is alcoholic or not. Menninger has said that alcoholism is a chronic form of suicide and, indeed, many alcoholics will so admit. There seem to be two settings for alcoholic suicide – impulsion and depression. Most suicide impulsively while intoxicated – alcohol being disinhibiting and depressing. Those alcoholics suiciding while depressed, either from the alcohol or other sources, have higher lethality and lower serotonin and 5-hydroxyindoleacetic acid in the cerebrospinal fluid.

30 Drinkers Who Are Not Alcoholics

Social drinking is a way of life for many and is not infrequently excessive in amount. The number of social drinkers with adverse consequences far exceeds the number of alcoholics. The amount consumed, the frequency of consumption and psychodynamics vary, but all are combined to lay the groundwork for psychosocial and health hazards.

Damages associated with ETOH abuse are generally more in the occupational and interpersonal areas than in physical health. Some of the common psychosocial consequencies are marital discord, personal embarrassment, absenteeism, blackouts, loss of friendships, belligerence, disinhibition of aggressive and sexual impulses, guilt feelings, ever-increasing denial, arrests, suicide, depression, financial difficulties. Health problems are fatty liver, elevated lipoproteins and cholesterol, hypertension, nutritional deficits and imbalances. There are increased risks for cardiovascular disease, esophageal cancer, cirrhosis, injury accidents, memory impairment, physiological dependence, and pancreatitis. Coronary disease has a J-shaped curve – small amounts of alcohol improve coronary flow but larger amounts reduce it. The risk of dependence is ever present.

While far from being precise and meant only to be general, Ray stated the following in reference to BAL: '30 mg/dl dull and dignified, 50 dashing and debonair, 100 dangerous and devilish, 200 dizzy and disturbing, 250 disturbing and disheveled, 300 delirious, disoriented and drunk, 350 dead drunk, 600 dead'.

One average drink contains approximately 20 g of alcohol. The chronic use of more than 80 g/day clearly risks health consequences. Ansties' limit (1870) for safe drinking is 1.5 oz of absolute alcohol per day (2 drinks) and probably still holds today. A safe guideline for any one occasion is an upper limit of 50 g for males and 35 g for females. For chronic use the upper safe limit should be 40 g for men and 25 g for women.

Even if those who drink to excess with adverse consequences do not progress to DSM-III alcoholism dependence, they still have psychopathology which should be treated. Reversal of pathology is often easier at this point and is usually preventive of progression to dependence. Physicians and the public need to take these matters as seriously as early cancer, diabetes or hypertension. The physician should take a good alcohol history from the patient and spouse, use the first 12 items on the MAST, and get a GTT when there is a high index of suspicion.

Recommended Reading

1   Alcoholics Anonymous. New York, AA World Services, 1939.
2   Anda RF, et al: Alcohol and fatal injuries among US adults. JAMA 1988;260:2529–2532.
3   Angur NA Jr: Gastric mucosal blood flow following damage by ethanol, acetic acid and or aspirin. Gastroenterology 1970;58:311.
4   Atkinson RM: Alcohol and Drug Abuse in Old Age. APPI, 1987.
5   Bean M, Zinberg N: Dynamic Approaches to the Understanding of Alcoholism. New York, Free Press, 1981.
6   Berglund M, Risberg J: Regional cerebral blood flow during alcohol withdrawal. Arch Gen Psychiatry 1981;38:351–355.
7   Bingham JR: Precipitating factors in peptic ulcer. Can Med Assoc J 1960;83:205.
8   Boulter BS: The effects of analgesics and anti-spasmodics on flow through the human common bile duct. Guys Hosp Rep 1961;110:246.
9   Bradus S, et al: Hepatic function and serum enzyme levels in association with fatty metamorphosis of the liver. Am J Med Sci 1963;245:35.
10 Burch ZE, Giles TD: Alcoholic cardiomyopathy. Biol Alcohol 1974;3:436–437.
11 Chang G, Astrachan B: The Emergency Department surveillance of alcohol intoxication after motor vehicle accidents. JAMA 1988;260:2533–2541.
12 Cleary P, et al: Prevalence and recognition of alcohol abuse in a primary care population. Am J Med 1988;85:466–471.
13 Craig JR, Mosier WM: Clinical and laboratory findings on admission to an alcohol detoxification service. Int J Addict 1978;13:1207–1215.
14 Davenport HW: Salicylate damage to the gastric mucosal barrier. N Engl J Med 1967;276:1307.
15 Eckhardt NJ, et al: Biochemical diagnosis of alcoholism. JAMA 1981;246:2707–2710.

16   Economou Z, Ward-McQuaid JN: A cross-over comparison of the effect of morphine, pethidine, pentazocine and phenazocine on biliary pressure. Gut 1971;12:218.

17   Ewing JA: Detecting alcoholism: The CAGE questionnaire. JAMA 1977;252:1905–1907.

18   Fisher C, Dement W: Studies in the psychopathology of sleep and dreams. Am J Psychiatry 1963;119:1160–1168.

19   Frances RJ, et al: Suicide and alcoholism. Am J Drug Alcohol Abuse 1987;13:327–341.

20   Frances RJ: Update on alcohol and drug disorder treatment. J Clin Psychiatry 1988;49(suppl):13–17.

21   Galanter M: Recent Developments in Alcoholism, vol I–IV. New York, Plenum Press, 1983–1986.

22   Galanter M, Pattison EM: Advances in the Psychosocial Treatment of Alcoholism. APPI, 1984.

23   Goldstein DB: Pharmacology of Alcoholism. Oxford, Oxford University Press, 1983.

24   Gresham SC, et al: Alcohol and caffeine: Effect on inferred visual dreaming. Science 1963;140:1226–1227.

25   Gross MM, et al: Experimental study of sleep in chronic alcoholics before, during and after 4 days of heavy drinking with a non-drinking companion. Ann NY Acad Sci 1973;215:254–265.

26   Harinasuta U, et al: Steatonecrosis: Mallory body type. Medicine 1967;46:141.

27   Helman RA, et al: Alcoholic hepatitis: Natural history and evaluation of prednisolone therapy. Ann Intern Med 1971;74:311.

28   Iber FL: Alcohol in the gastrointestinal tract. Gastroenterology 1971;61:120.

29   Kaufman E: Substance Abuse and Family Therapy. New York, Grune & Stratton, 1985.

30   Kissin B, Begleiter H: The Biology of Acoholism, vol I–VII. New York, Plenum Press, 1971–1983.

31   Kewenter J, Kock NG: The effect of some spasmolytic drugs on the choledochoduodenal junction in man. Scand J Gastroenterol 1971; 6:401.

32   Klion FM, Rudavsky F: False positive liver scans in patients with alcoholic liver disease. Am J Intern Med 1968;69:283.

33   Knott DH: Guidelines for diagnosis and alcohol detoxification. Drug Ther 1978:35–47.

34   Knott DH, et al: Intoxication and the alcohol abstinence syndrome. Postgrad Med 1981;69:65–69, 72–75.

35   Koegel P, Burnam A: Alcoholism among homeless adults in the inner city of Los Angeles. Arch Gen Psychiatry 1988;45:1011–1018.

36 Laurie JA: Gin and the sickle cell crisis. Lancet 1971;i:1354.

37 Lindenbaum J: Hematologic effects of alcohol. Biol Alcohol 1974; 3:461–480.

38 Lyons HA, Sultzman A: Diseases of the respiratory tract in alcoholics. Biol Alcohol 1974;3:406.

39 Mendelson J, Mello N: The Diagnosis and Treatment of Alcoholism. New York, McGraw-Hill, 1985.

40 Meyer RE, Kranzler HR: Alcoholism: Clinical implications of recent research. J Clin Psychiatry 1988;49(suppl):8–12.

41 Miria SN: Substance Abuse and Psychopathology. APPI, 1984.

42 Monteiro MG, Schuckit M: Populations at high alcoholism risk: Recent findings. J Clin Psychiatry 1988;49(suppl):8–12.

43 Pattison EM, Kaufman E: Encyclopedic Handbook of Alcoholism. New York, Gardner Press, 1982.

44 Pirola RC, Lieber CS: Acute and chronic pancreatitis. Biol Alcohol 1974;3:385–388.

45 Pokorny AD, et al: The brief MAST: A shortened version of the Michigan Alcoholism Screening Test. Am J Psychiatry 1972;129: 342–345.

46 Rankin JZ, et al: Relationship between smoking and pulmonary disease in alcoholism. Med J Aust 1969;i:730–733.

47 Ratnoff OD, Patdek AJ: The natural history of Laennec's cirrhosis of the liver. Medicine 1942;21:207.

48 Robertson CB, Sellers EM: Alcohol intoxication and the alcohol withdrawal syndrome. Postgrad Med 1978;64:133–138.

48 Roine RP, et al: Serum acetate as a marker of problem drinking among drunken drivers. Alcohol Alcohol 1988;23:123–126.

49 Rose HB, et al: Causes of fever in alcoholics in withdrawal. Am J Med Sci 1970;260:112–121.

49 Rothermich NA, von Hamm E: Pancreatic encephalopathy. J Clin Endocrinol 1941;1:1892.

50 Schuckit MA: Drug and Alcohol Abuse, ed 2. New York, Plenum Press, 1984.

51 Schuckit MA, Irwin M: Diagnosis of alcoholism. Med Clin North Am 1988;72:1133–1153.

52 Shader RJ, Greenblatt D: Manual of Psychiatric Therapeutics. Boston, Little Brown, 1975.

53 Solomon J: Alcohol and Clinical Psychiatry. New York, Plenum Press, 1982.

54 Vaillant G: The Natural History of Alcoholism. Cambridge, Harvard University Press, 1983.

55 Valaske MJ: Laboratory clues suggesting alcoholism. Md State Med J 1980;29:59–61.

56   Victor M, Brausch C: The role of abstinence in the genesis of alcoholic epilepsy. Epilepsia 1967;8:1–20.

57   Victor M: The role of hypomagnesemia and respiratory alkalosis in the genesis of alcohol withdrawal syndrome. Ann NY Acad Sci 1973;215:235–248.

58   Weiss AD, et al: Experimentally induced chronic intoxication and withdrawal in alcoholics. Q J Stud Alcohol 1964;(suppl 2):24.

59   Westermeyer J, Neider J: Social networks and psychopathology among substance abusers. Am J Psychiatry 1988;145:1265–1269.

60   Wolfe SM, et al: Respiratory alkalosis and alcohol withdrawal. Trans Assoc Am Physicians 1969;82:344–352.

61   Wollman H, et al: Effect of respiratory and metabolic alkalosis on cerebral blood flow in man. J Appl Physiol 1968;24:60–65.

62   Zimberg S: The Clinical Management of Alcoholism. New York, Brunner/Mazel, 1982.

63   Zimberg S, Wallace J, Blume S: Practical Approaches to Alcoholism Psychotherapy. New York, Plenum Press, 1985.

Subject Index